ONCE UPON A TIME, IN A LIVELY LITTLE TOWN, LIVED TWO ADVENTUROUS FRIENDS Max and Sophie

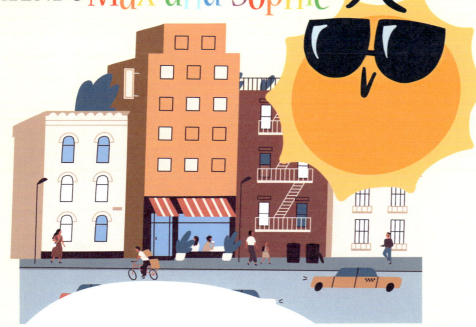

THEY LOVED EXPLORING THEIR NEIGHBORHOOD AND GOING ON EXCITING ADVENTURES.

ONE SUNNY DAY, THEY DECIDED TO WALK TO THEIR FAVORITE PARK, BUT TO GET THERE, THEY HAD TO CROSS A BUSY STREET.

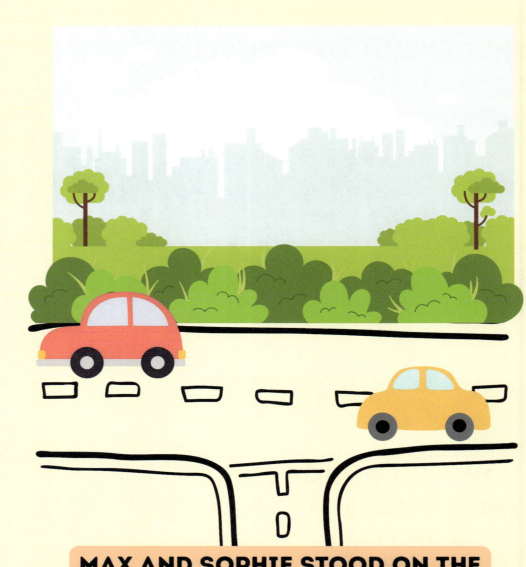

MAX AND SOPHIE STOOD ON THE SIDEWALK, LOOKING AT THE CARS ZOOMING PAST. THEY KNEW THEY HAD TO BE CAREFUL AND CROSS THE STREET SAFELY. THEY REMEMBERED THE IMPORTANT TIPS THEIR PARENTS HAD TAUGHT THEM ABOUT STREET CROSSING.

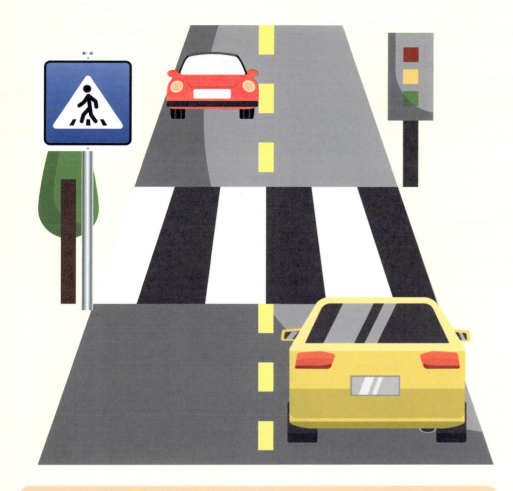

THE FIRST THING MAX AND SOPHIE DID WAS FIND A DESIGNATED CROSSING AREA. THEY SPOTTED A ZEBRA CROSSING A SHORT DISTANCE AWAY. THEY KNEW IT WAS A SAFE SPOT TO CROSS BECAUSE DRIVERS WERE REQUIRED TO STOP AND LET PEDESTRIANS CROSS.

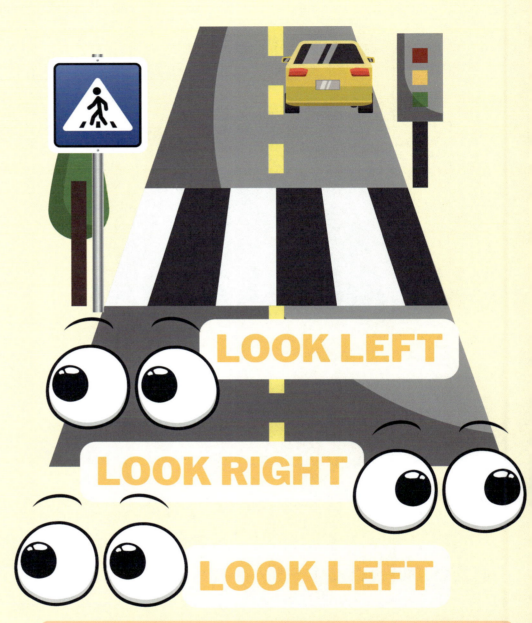

LOOK LEFT

LOOK RIGHT

LOOK LEFT

BEFORE STEPPING ONTO THE ZEBRA CROSSING, MAX AND SOPHIE REMEMBERED TO LOOK LEFT, RIGHT, AND LEFT AGAIN. THEY KNEW IT WAS IMPORTANT TO CHECK FOR ANY ONCOMING CARS, BICYCLES, OR MOTORCYCLES. THEY WAITED FOR A CLEAR GAP IN THE TRAFFIC BEFORE PROCEEDING.

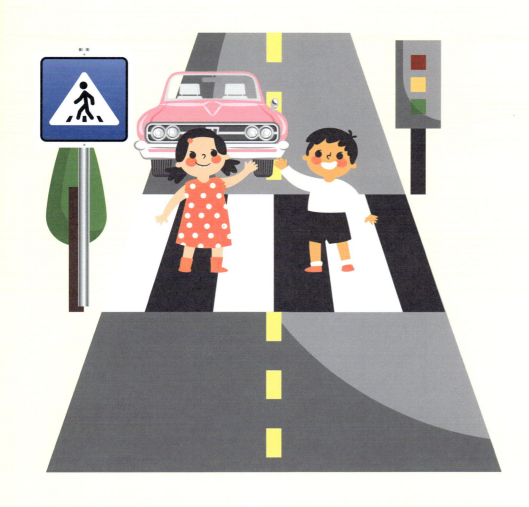

ONCE THEY MADE SURE IT WAS SAFE, MAX AND SOPHIE STEPPED ONTO THE ZEBRA CROSSING. THEY WALKED CALMLY AND STEADILY, MAKING SURE TO STAY WITHIN THE LINES. THEY KNEW IT WAS IMPORTANT NOT TO RUSH OR RUN ACROSS THE STREET, AS IT COULD BE DANGEROUS.

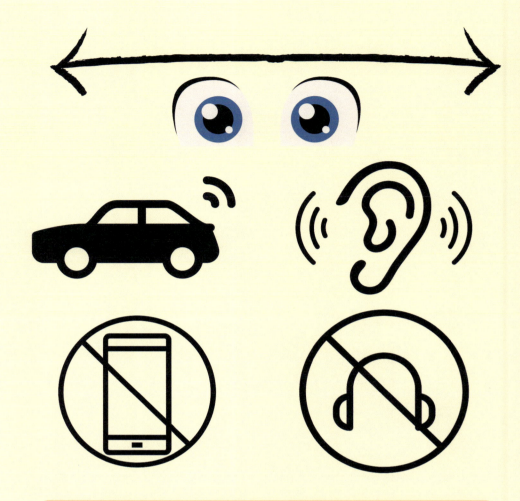

AS MAX AND SOPHIE CROSSED THE STREET, THEY KEPT THEIR EYES AND EARS OPEN. THEY KNEW THEY SHOULD BE AWARE OF ANY UNEXPECTED SOUNDS OR MOVEMENTS. THEY ALSO AVOIDED DISTRACTIONS, SUCH AS USING THEIR PHONES OR LISTENING TO MUSIC, AS IT COULD MAKE THEM LESS AWARE OF THEIR SURROUNDINGS.

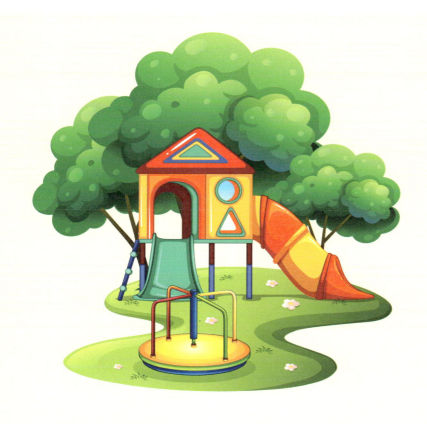

MAX AND SOPHIE REACHED THE OTHER SIDE OF THE STREET SAFELY. THEY FELT ACCOMPLISHED AND PROUD OF THEMSELVES FOR CROSSING THE STREET RESPONSIBLY. THEY KNEW THAT BY FOLLOWING THE SAFETY GUIDELINES, THEY HAD MADE IT TO THE PARK WITHOUT ANY HARM.

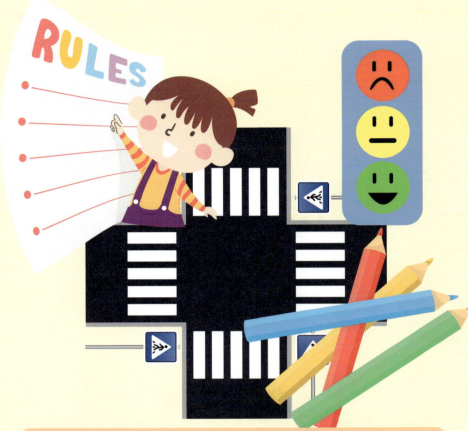

MAX AND SOPHIE REALIZED THE IMPORTANCE OF STREET SAFETY AND DECIDED TO SHARE THEIR KNOWLEDGE WITH THEIR FRIENDS. THEY WANTED EVERYONE TO KNOW HOW TO CROSS THE STREET SAFELY. THEY ORGANIZED A SMALL WORKSHOP AT SCHOOL, WHERE THEY TAUGHT THEIR FRIENDS THE TIPS FOR A SAFE STREET CROSSING.

RULES

RULES

RULES

RULES

#1
FINDING A SAFE SPOT

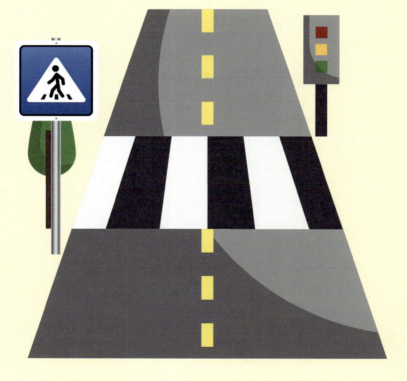

#2
LOOK LEFT, RIGHT, AND LEFT AGAIN

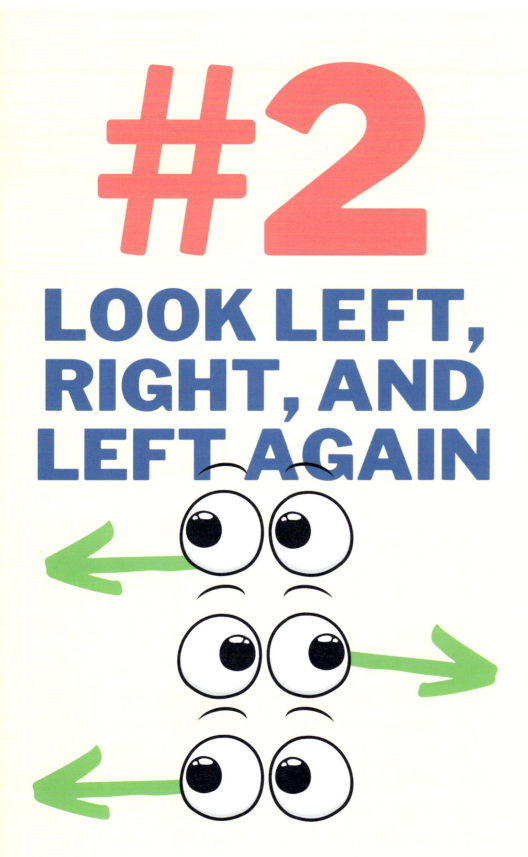

#3

WALKING ACROSS THE STREET

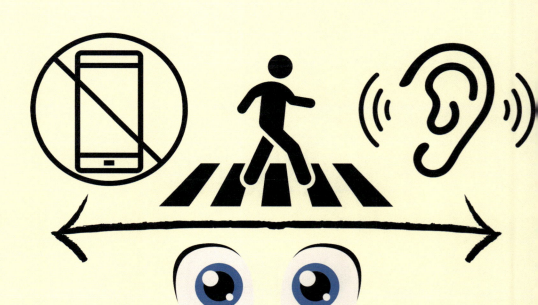

#5

ASK FOR HELP

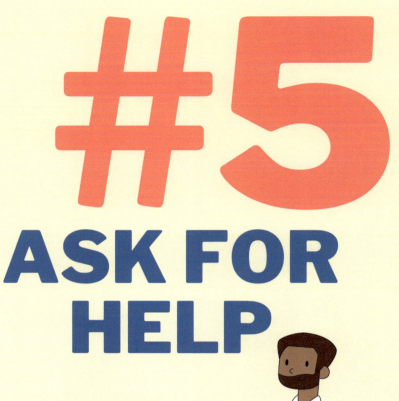

IF POSSIBLE, ASK AN ADULT FOR HELP WHEN CROSSING THE STREET.

GREAT!
YOU HAVE LEARNED SOME VERY IMPORTANT RULES. LET'S SEE IF YOU REMEMBER HOW TO CROSS THE STREET SAFELY.

CHOOSE A SAFER PLACE
TO CROSS THE STREET

#1

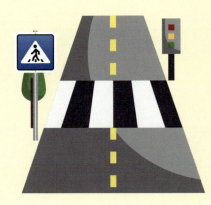

#2

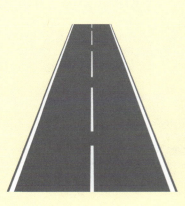

HOW DO WE MAKE SURE IF WE CAN CROSS THE STREET?

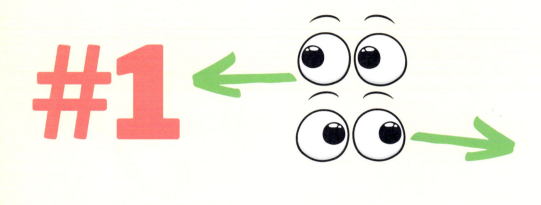

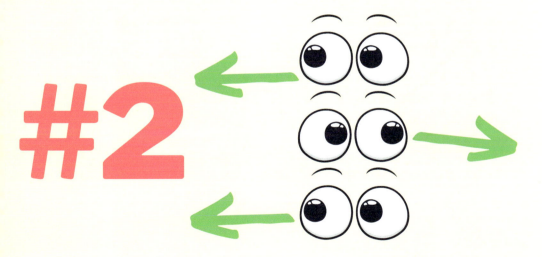

POINT OUT WHAT YOU MUST NOT DO WHILE CROSSING THE STREET

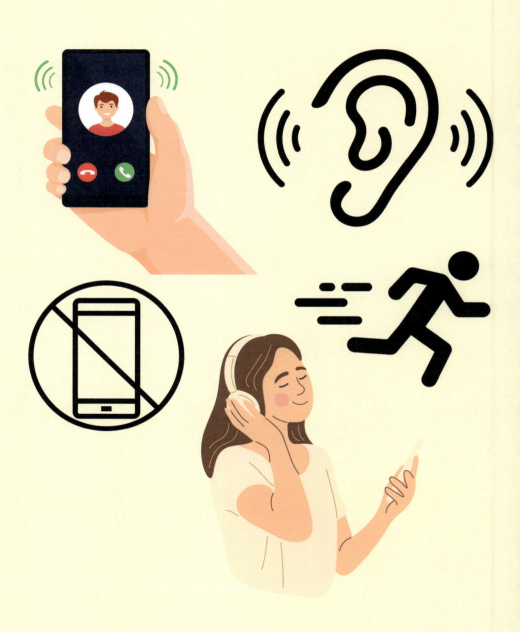

IF THERE IS A TRAFFIC LIGHT, ON WHICH LIGHT CAN WE CROSS THE STREET?

#1

#2

THE MOST IMPORTANT SIGNS AND SIGNALS.

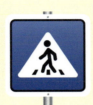

THE PEDESTRIAN CROSSING SIGN

ZEBRA CROSSING.

PEDESTRIAN SIGNAL LIGHTS

GREAT!
TEACH YOUR FRIENDS TO FOLLOW THE RULES ON THE STREET, AND EVERYONE WILL REACH THEIR DESTINATION SAFELY!

COLOR THE PICTURE

COLOR THE PICTURE

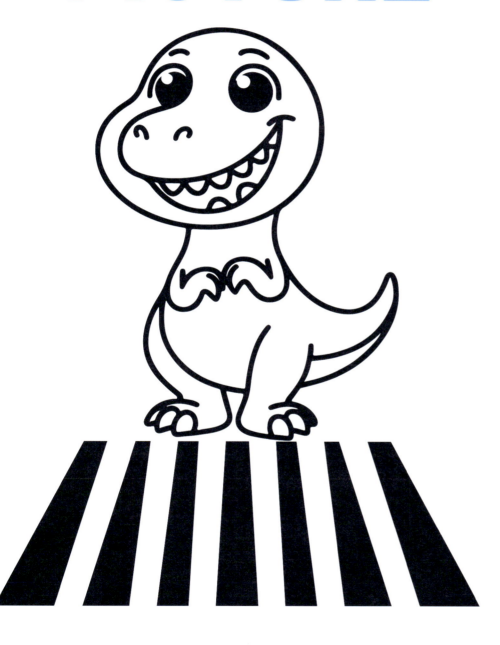

COLOR THE PICTURE

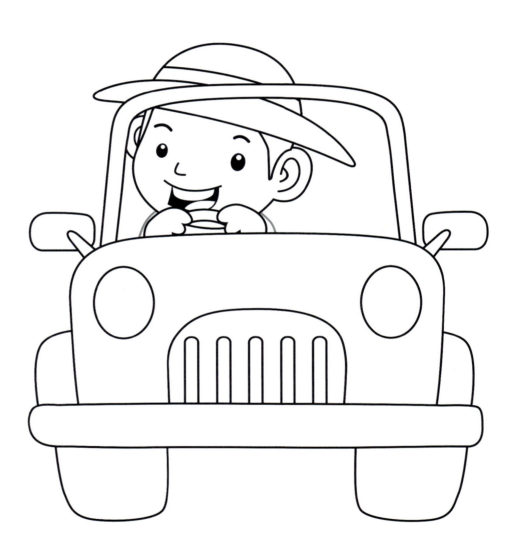

Made in United States
Troutdale, OR
04/06/2025

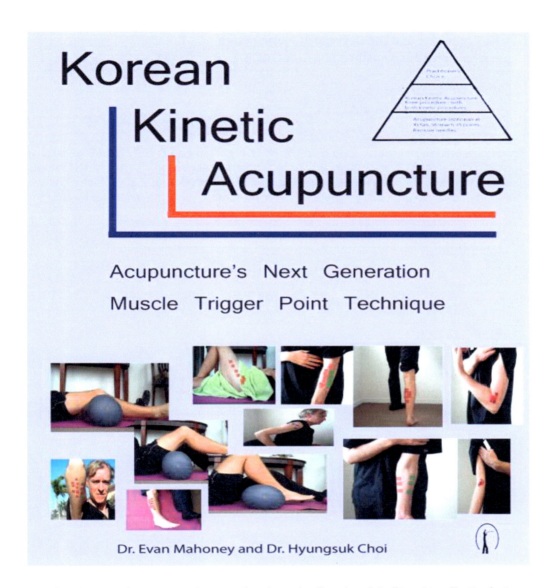

Korean Kinetic Acupuncture

Acupuncture's Next Generation

Muscle Trigger Point Technique

Dr. Evan Mahoney and Dr. Hyungsuk Choi

This hardcopy edition contains two books. The first book is "Dry Needle Technique and Arguments for the Defense of Acupuncture". The second book is "Korean Kinetic Acupuncture"

Dry Needle Technique and the Defense of Acupuncture
VST Acupuncture, Capstone and Credentials

By Dr. Evan Mahoney
Copyright 2015

I wrote this for three reasons, all of which have to do with 'credentials'.

1. There was a private criticism made of my school Samra University and myself (through affiliation with school), during the writing of "Arguments for the Defense of Acupuncture".   This is my response.
2. To pre-eminently establish Kinetic Acupuncture and its components mentioned in this (and my other books) as pre-eminent acupuncture techniques, pedigreed and derived from Acupuncture and Korea.
3. Additional document as a source of curriculum for dry needle in the lexicon of acupuncture.

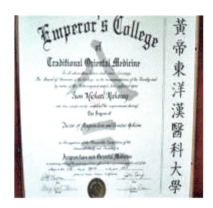

In 2009 I was in the gust of the greatest professional moment of my life, accepted under salary and scholarship into Samra University's, Samra Acupuncture Center Doctoral Program. I worked and studied full time learning and practicing Korean Acupuncture techniques for the treatment of pain. The techniques included were Korean Kinetic Acupuncture, Isometric, Tuina Stretching, VST Acupuncture (which is the subject and study of my doctoral capstone presented here), and Saam Acupuncture (which was in continuation of my previous six years study with Dr. Tao Cheong Choo, the first and foremost Saam instructor in America and Europe).

It was through relationships forged during completion of my masters degree in Acupuncture and Oriental Medicine and in my interview where my ideas on meditation and marketing corresponded with Dr. Choi's conceptions that I got hired. I was one of four out of 100 applicants who were accepted into the program.

With twenty treatment rooms, a half million dollar MRI imaging center, four branches in California and New Jersey, the financial support of Hamsoa Children's Hospital and a plan for growth and expansion I was hired to learn the techniques of Samra Acupuncture Center and teach them in new clinics across the country.

It was a great time. In Samra Acupuncture Center's Los Angeles Branch we treated celebrities, athletes, and the general public, seeing over 100 patients a day, amongst three chief practitioners and support staff. We had networking lunches and visits to Koreatown business owners, regular dinners and lectures amongst staff. I worked and studied at Dr. Choi's side for a year and a half. During this time we forged a similar dream of America and 100 clinics.

Abruptly the program and school shut down. It was the decision of President Park, lawyer and owner of Samra University and Abraham Lincoln Law School. I am unsure of the clinic's financial obligations at the time. I do not think that was the reason for declaring bankruptcy. I believe it may have been done to get out of a long term lease commitment made with the landlord whom President Park had a dispute with. Bankruptcy was a poor decision on his part. Dr. Choo would have been ready to take over the school had President Park consulted with him. Instead bankruptcy was declared and the school lost its accreditation. Dr. Choo did buy Samra out of bankruptcy and may still to this day have plans to revive accreditation. The lives of those invested in Samra's program were touched and I feel sadness at our dispersion. I consider my books and work to be a continuing completion of the mission that I was hired for.

In 2011 I completed my doctorate at Emperor's College with endearing gratefulness to the late Academic Dean, David Migocki who accepted our cohort from Samra's Doctoral program.

****

The subject of my capstone is on VST acupuncture (Vertex Synchronizing Technique) created by Dr. Jonghwa Lee who ran Samra Acupuncture Center's branch clinic in Irvine. VST acupuncture was practiced in our clinic along side of Korean Kinetic Acupuncture which is a technique created by my teacher Dr. Hyungsuk Choi. VST is an acupuncture equivalent of the Dry Needle Technique.

I was not aware in 2011 (when I co-wrote my capstone paper with my fellow researchers) of the controversy that would build surrounding Dry Needle as Physical Therapist, Chiropractors and others try to incorporate this technique into their procedures.

The techniques presented here and in my other books may have attempts made in the future to be pre-empted upon and declared in terms like Kinetic Dry Needle, or Kinetic Dry Needling. It is my intent here to firmly declare that the technique and components pertaining to Korean Kinetic Acupuncture originate from Acupuncture and Korea. Korean Kinetic Acupuncture and its components are pre-eminent acupuncture techniques.

Many of the techniques practiced at Samra Acupuncture Center are written about in my other books, in particular "Saam Korean Acupuncture: Advanced Combinations". My "Fountain of Youth Stretch Series" is also derived from my experience at Samra Acupuncture Center's clinic.

My Credentials:

These books form some of my credentials derived from the great program, faculty, and staff involved with Samra University and Samra Acupuncture Center.

Saam Meditation/ Acupuncture

Five (e) - Book Series by Dr. Evan Mahoney

Available at Amazon.com

Fountain of Youth Stretching

Two (e)-Book & Video Series by Dr. Evan Mahoney

Available at Amazon.com

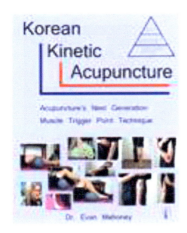

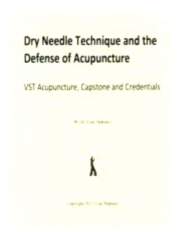

Samra Acupuncture Center Brochure - Los Angeles CA 2009

Written by Dr. Choi and I. We thought long about what to call our technique. I came up with the term Mobility Plus, which is meant as an all inclusive term for the multiple techniques we practiced.

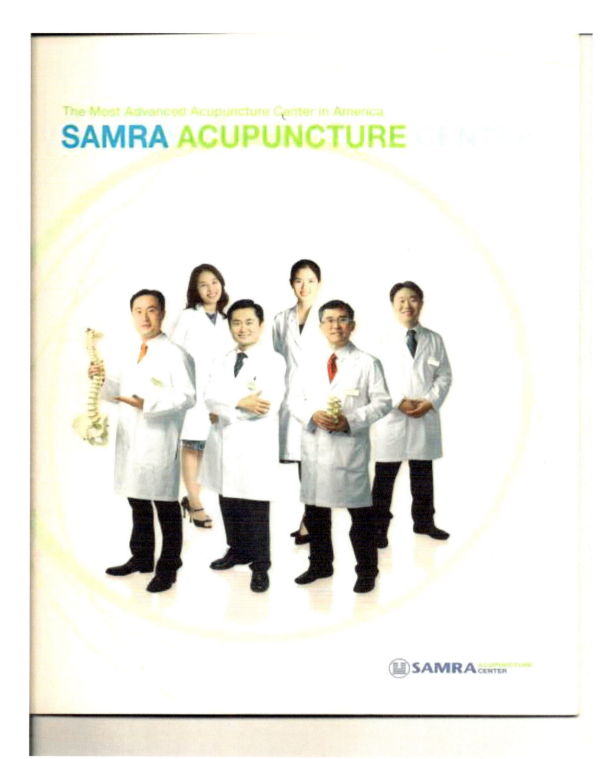

Figure 1 Dr. Hyungsuk Choi, center Left. Dr. Jonghwa Lee far right

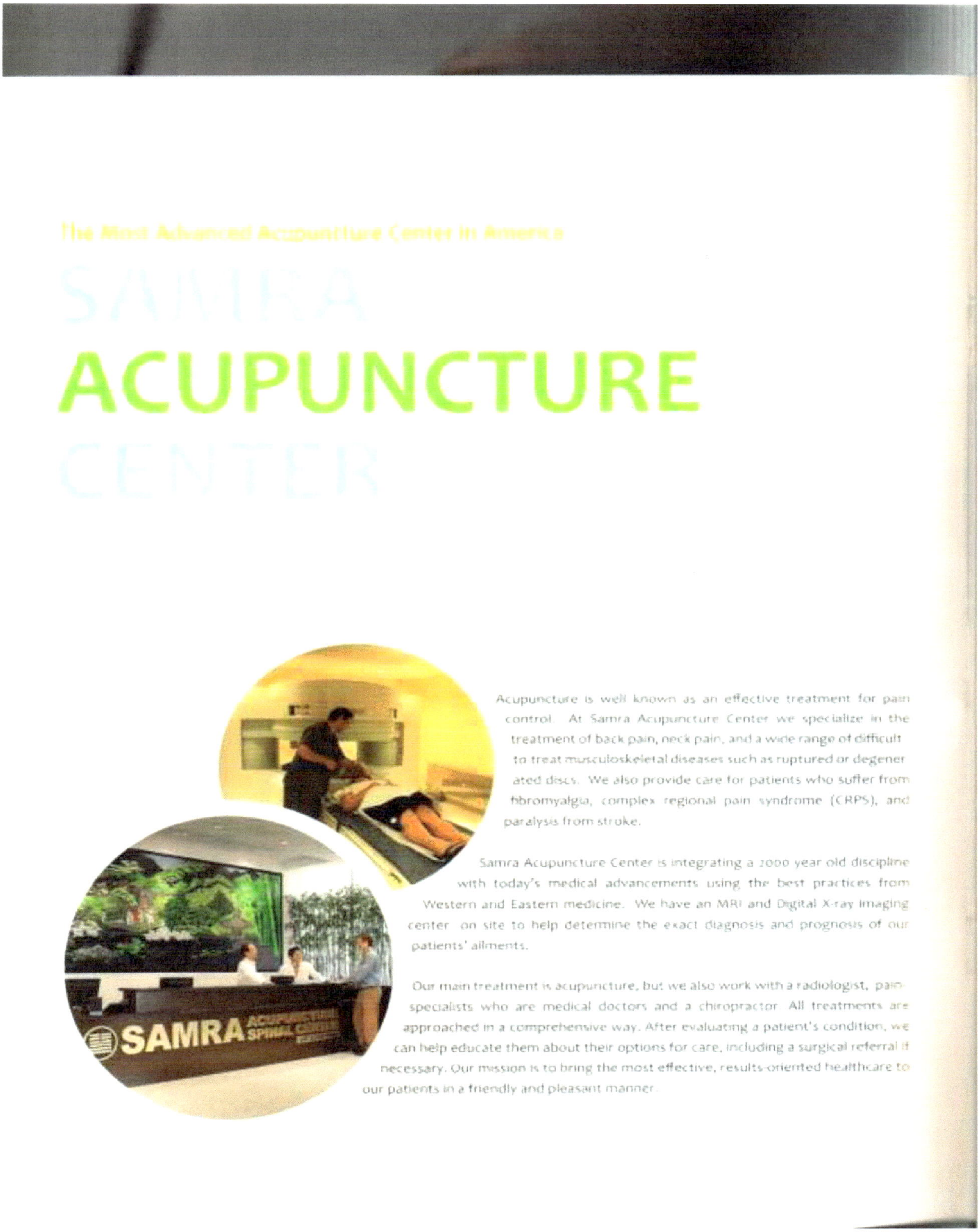

The Most Advanced Acupuncture Center in America

SAMRA

ACUPUNCTURE

CENTER

Acupuncture is well known as an effective treatment for pain control. At Samra Acupuncture Center we specialize in the treatment of back pain, neck pain, and a wide range of difficult to treat musculoskeletal diseases such as ruptured or degenerated discs. We also provide care for patients who suffer from fibromyalgia, complex regional pain syndrome (CRPS), and paralysis from stroke.

Samra Acupuncture Center is integrating a 2000 year old discipline with today's medical advancements using the best practices from Western and Eastern medicine. We have an MRI and Digital X-ray imaging center on site to help determine the exact diagnosis and prognosis of our patients' ailments.

Our main treatment is acupuncture, but we also work with a radiologist, pain specialists who are medical doctors and a chiropractor. All treatments are approached in a comprehensive way. After evaluating a patient's condition, we can help educate them about their options for care, including a surgical referral if necessary. Our mission is to bring the most effective, results-oriented healthcare to our patients in a friendly and pleasant manner.

Figure 2 Really appreciating and remembering the artwork we left behind on that wall.

Many Korean celebrities came to our clinic, as well as professional and collegiate athletes. I am in the picture with a couple of foot ball players third row down fourth picture to the left.

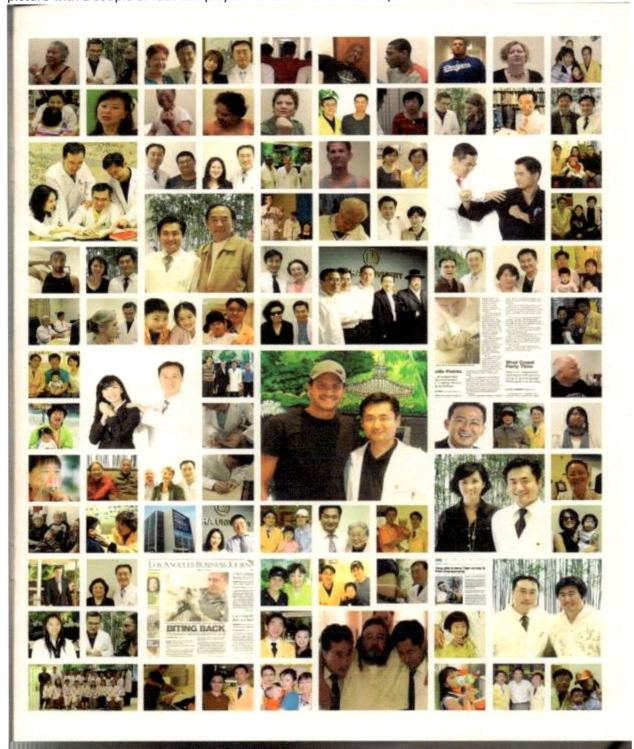

Our World Class Doctors Make the Difference.

Samra clinics offer specialized acupuncture services, based upon years of scientific research and experience. Our physicians and specialists are leaders in their fields. The training of acupuncturists in Korea is quite rigorous, requiring ten years of academic study, internship, and residency. In fact, Korean Oriental medical schools are as selective and competitive to enter as conventional medical schools. Our doctors are at the top of their class and profession.

Key Seung Gwak, DC, LAc
(Professor of Oriental Medicine, Samra University)

- California Licensed Acupuncturist
- California Licensed Chiropractor
- NCCAOM Diplomate Acupuncture & Herbology
- D.C. Cleveland Chiropractic College
- Diplomate California Chiropractic Board
- Member of American Chiropractic Association
- Member of California Chiropractic Association
- Radiography Supervisor and Operator Permit, California

Hyungsuk Choi, CEO, PhD, LAc
(Professor of Oriental Medicine, Samra University)

- PhD, MS, Complementary and Alternative Medicine College of Medicine, Pochon CHA University
- B.A. Oriental Medicine, Kyung Hee University
- Researcher, Department of Herbology, Kyung Hee University
- Staff Physician (Oriental Medicine), Public Health Center
- Staff Physician (Oriental Medicine), Jangsu Oriental Medical Center
- Professional course of alternative medicine for cancer, Pochon CHA Univ. Graduate school of CAM
- Intern and Resident with Specialty of Acupuncture at Bosaeng, Oriental Medical Center
- Editor of Korean Oriental Association for Study of Obesity

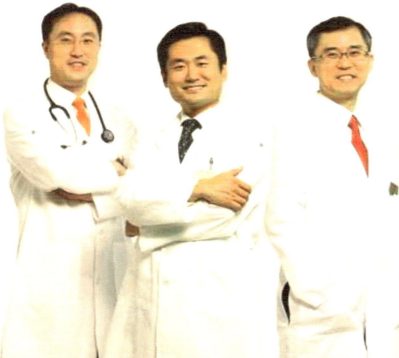

Kiwan Ko, PhD, LAc
(Professor of Oriental Medicine, Samra University)

- PhD, MS, Oriental Medicine, Kyung Hee University
- MS, Public Health Policy & Management, Yonsei University
- PhD, MS, Complementary and Alternative Medicine, Pochon CHA University
- Certificate from Executive CEO Education Program for Public Health Management, Seoul National University, Korea and School of Public Health at Harvard University, Boston, MA
- CEO & President, Kwangdong Oriental Medical Hospital
- Adjunct Professor, Dongbang, Pochon CHA & Sanggi University
- Lecturer, Oriental Medicine, Aju, Seoul Women's College of Nursing, Daegu Haany & Kyung Hee University

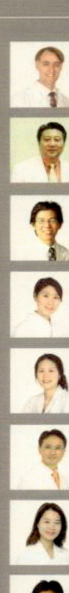
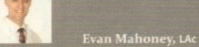

Evan Mahoney, LAc

- B.A, University of Pittsburgh, Pennsylvania
- M.A, Oriental Medicine, Samra University of Oriental Medicine
- Current Resident Doctor, Samra Acupuncture Center/ DAOM program
- California licensed acupuncturist
- Diplomat in oriental medicine (NCCAOM)

Philip Doh, MD

- Yonsei Pain Clinic, Specializing in Pain Management
- Medical Director for Pain Clinic and Anesthesia Department
- State University of New York Health Science Center at Brooklyn
- Yonsei University College of Medicine
- Board Certification: American Board of Anesthesiology

PalKeun Song, LAc

- O.M.D, University of Yanbian, China
- Staff Physician, Hanuoo Children's Clinic of Oriental Medicine
- Staff Physician, Yeol-Un Acupuncture Clinic
- Staff Physician, Acu Chiro Clinic
- California licensed acupuncturist
- Diplomat in oriental medicine (NCCAOM)

Heejoo Kim, LAc

- B.A., Molecular and Cell Biology, University of California at Berkeley, CA
- M.A, Oriental Medicine, Southern California University, CA
- California licensed acupuncturist
- Current Resident Doctor, Samra Acupuncture Center/ DAOM program
- Staff practitioner, Asian Health Services, Oakland, CA
- Staff, Southern California University of Health Science, Whittier, CA

Minkyung Oh, LAc

- B.A, Sahm Yook University, Korea
- M.A, Oriental Medicine, Samra University of Oriental Medicine
- Current Resident Doctor, Samra Acupuncture Center/ DAOM program
- California licensed acupuncturist

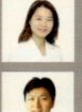

Juho Park, LAc

- M.A, Seoul National University, Korea
- M.A, Oriental Medicine, Samra University of Oriental Medicine
- Current Resident Doctor, Samra Acupuncture Center/ DAOM program
- City of Los Angeles licensed massage therapist
- Staff practitioner, Hospice at Bergen Community Health Care, NJ
- Staff practitioner, Care Alternatives, Hospice for the Life We Live, NJ

Renee Ahn,

- B.A, Ajou University, Korea
- California & New York licensed Nurse
- Current Intern, Samra Acupuncture Center/ M.A program
- Staff RN, Ajou University Hospital, Korea
- Licensed Nurse and Midwife, Korea
- Licensed sport massage therapist, Korea

Shawn YangRN

- B.A, Cal State University in San Bernadino, CA
- M.S, Cal State University in San Bernadino, CA
- Scholarship student in South Baylo University, CA
- Current Intern, Samra Acupuncture Center/ M.A program

Drew E.Fenton, MD

- Board Certification and Re-Certification by the American Board of Emergency Medicine
- Residency training in Emergency Medicine at University of Southern California Medical Center
- Internship Internal Medicine, Letterman Army Medical Center, San Francisco, CA
- MD, Thomas Jefferson Medical College, Philadelphia, PA
- Elected to the Board of Directors and as Secretary/ Treasurer of the American Academy of Emergency Medicine.

Inside Samra Acupuncture Center

At Samra Acupuncture Center, we take a multi-disciplinary approach to assess your mild discipline to...

Contemporary Diagnostic Tools

Unlike most acupuncture clinics which rely on questionnaires as their diagnostic tools, Samra Acupuncture Center utilizes state-of-the-art Magnetic Resonance Imaging (MRI), Nerve Conduction Velocity (NCV), and Digital X Ray imaging to help us accurately pinpoint the origin of our patients' symptoms. We believe this is a crucial part of the acupuncture process, not only because it provides the clearest diagnoses, but it also rules out any life-threatening conditions which might require immediate medical intervention. At Samra Acupuncture Center, medical doctors, chiropractors and acupuncturists all work together, so that the patients' diagnoses and care are viewed from a comprehensive perspective.

Mobility + Acupuncture

"Keep your arms swinging, one-two, one-two, and one-two," leads the instructor as a young man performs what appears to be a formal and vigorous military march. This man is not in training for the army. He is being treated for back pain. If you look closely, you can see that he has barely visible acupuncture needles in his arms and legs. This is part of Samra Acupuncture Center's 'Mobility plus Acupuncture'. This unique treatment of needles and movement has helped alleviate severe and acute pain in many of our patients. Most patients experience immediate and extreme relief.

Our treatments deliver
- Pain relief
- Optimal function
- Balanced structure

Alignment

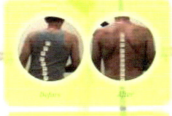

Structure + Function

Structure Balancing With Acupuncture

Mobility

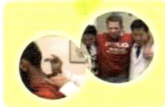

Passive & Active Exercise With Acupuncture

The Concept Behind
Mobility + Acupuncture

The body has both structure (**yin**) and function (**yang**); they are two sides of a coin. The human body should be treated as a whole, encompassing both aspects.

Structure

The human spine is like a mast on a sailboat. In order for the mast to be stable and upright, it must be sustained by many ropes. When we treat a patient's back pain, we do not work directly on the spine (**mast**), but rather on the muscles (**ropes**) attached to it. By using acupuncture, we can balance the tension of muscles and eventually obtain the proper stance of the spine.

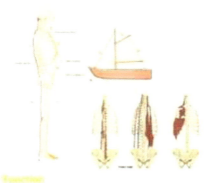

Function

In order to promote optimal function, we induce passive and active movements while needles are in place. Needles act to clear and dredge the blockages that can occur in muscles, joints or nerves. Active motion with needles in place improves the circulation of blood and oxygen to the area. This, in turn, helps to improve lubrication between tissues and promote healing.

Patients walk with needles or perform special workouts designed for their individual injury. In conventional acupuncture, the needles are inserted and the patient remains static. 'Mobility plus Acupuncture' treats the human body as a dynamic, moving entity.

Common Pains Treated by
Mobility + Acupuncture

The doctors at Samra Acupuncture Center use 'Mobility plus Acupuncture' for a wide variety of symptoms. In the treatment of lower back, shoulder, elbow, wrist or knee pain, the doctor will induce passive and active movements, while the needles are in place. This allows the doctor to stimulate the end of the joint cavity and all the muscles attached to the joint. Frozen shoulder patients who couldn't move their arms have been able to get dressed, lift their arms, and touch the opposite ear after just a few treatments.

At Samra Acupuncture Center, We Treat;

- **Spine related disorders**
  - Low back pain, neck pain, sciatica
  - Disc problems
  - Post surgical pain
- **Musculoskeletal pain**
  - Acute and chronic pain unresponsive to other treatments (Physical therapies, chiropractic care, epidural injections, etc.)
  - Doctors/ Patients want to explore a different approach
- **Workplace injuries (workers compensation)**
- **Personal injuries (traffic accidents)**
  - Treatment of unspecified pain
  - Restoration of function
- **Fibromyalgia**
- **Chronic fatigue syndrome**
- **Complex Regional Pain Syndrome**
- **Frozen shoulder / Impingement syndrome**
- **Knee complaints**

Covered by Major Insurance !

Call or Visit for Insurance verification

213-384-1100   www.samraclinic.com
1730 W. Olympic Blvd., Suite 100, Los Angeles, CA 90015

GLOBAL
ACUPUNCTURE

Beyond Korea and around the world.
We provide superior acupuncture treatment.

From our first acupuncture center in Korea, SAMRA has expanded to become a world leader in Oriental Medicine. Our goal is to establish more than 100 branches in the United States of America, so that our patients can visit Samra Acupuncture Centers throughout the country.

SAMRA Affiliations

 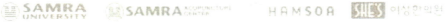

USA

SAMRA operates clinics under the name of Hamsoa, She's Clinic, and Samra Acupuncture Center in the United States. Thus far, we have four locations- Los Angeles and Fullerton, California, New York, and New Jersey.

CHINA

SAMRA operating under the name 'Hamsoa' in Asia, has a branch in Shanghai with plans for adding more branches throughout China.

021.5058.7990

KOREA

Hamsoa is the most successful Oriental Medicine Clinic in Korea for treating children, with over 51 branches throughout the country. Koreans can visit a Hamsoa clinic anywhere in the nation. For over ten years, mothers have come to trust the care their children receive at Hamsoa clinics.
We have also recently opened a pharmaceutical company, producing the finest quality herbal medicines for both children and adults.

82.1544.1075

Los Angeles
213.384.1100

Fullerton
714.562.7000

New York
718.939.6700

New Jersey
201.592.9800

SAMRA UNIVERSITY OF ORIENTAL MEDICINE

Samra University, a private, non-profit corporation, is the oldest school of Oriental Medicine in the United States. In 1969, we became the first school of Oriental Medicine to receive Full Institutional Approval by the California State Department of Education. Our Master of Oriental Medicine Degree program is accredited by the Accreditation Commission for Acupuncture and Oriental Medicine. Samra University of Oriental Medicine is known internationally as a premiere teaching institution. Our reputation draws students from throughout the world. To accommodate students' varying backgrounds, classes are taught separately in three languages: English, Mandarin Chinese and Korean.

213.381.2221

Youtube videos made at Samra Acupuncture Center

https://www.youtube.com/watch?v=YGtz1_BhFYc - Me with back pain patient.

https://www.youtube.com/watch?v=MZJhIkhjJ4k - Dr. Choi is presented. I filmed and conducted interview.

https://www.youtube.com/watch?v=RV0J5s_cGKM - Samra Acupuncture Center's TV commercial aired on cable TV.

https://www.youtube.com/watch?v=6UKow7YFbHw - Me interviewing Dr. Choo - Saam Acupuncture.

https://www.youtube.com/watch?v=S21glL-s7hY - Me interviewing Dr. Jonghwa lee on VST Acupuncture.

Youtube videos accompanying the study of this book.

https://www.youtube.com/watch?v=VsjICmX0Yrs&t=0s - Part 1
https://www.youtube.com/watch?v=dXvDgOGPS2s   - Part 2
https://www.youtube.com/watch?v=5hBbcifIAus   - Part 3
https://www.youtube.com/watch?v=MIcm1WSS0HM   - Part 4

Articles on Acupuncture's Dry Needle Technique

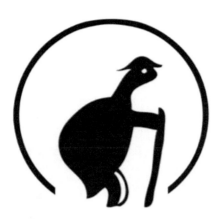

3.15.15

Arguments for the Defense of Acupuncture and its Related Modalities and Procedures

Goals of publishing the statement "Arguments for the Defense of Acupuncture and its Related Modalities and Procedures"

1. To Firmly Re-Assert Acupuncture Physiology as Science

2. To Firmly Declare the Preeminence of the Language of Acupuncture

3. To document the Dry Needle Technique Expansion into Identical Pre-eminent Acupuncture Techniques

4. To mathematically document in the Physical Therapists own logic, the current insufficient education practices in training of Dry Needle Technique.

Arguments for the Defense of Acupuncture and its Related Modalities and Procedures

We acupuncturist, licensed in Acupuncture and Oriental Medicine, notice a grave threat and recognize an obligation to uphold the traditions of acupuncture and its related modalities to a standard worthy of their greatest dignity, maturity, and respect.

We are concerned regarding the use, procedures, safety, and public ethical problems associated with the too-fast, too-loosely-regulated, and too-insufficiently trained practices of Acupuncture's increasing usage within Physical Therapy, Chiropractic, and others business and clinical settings. There is insufficient training, knowledge, and time of study involved in such practices. Consequently, these practitioners are unable to competently and ethically interact in clinical, private, and public settings involving acupuncture and its associated modalities.

We believe the current allowable training practices of a minimum of 27[i]- 46 hours[ii] (with variance among states) needed to practice dry needle to be insufficient. It renders one quick to action, quick to practice, and quick to believe in one's own competency[iii], without the underlying foundations of knowledge and experience. It is also a risk to public health and safety.

We also assert that the Physical Therapy community is on course to expand the scope of dry needle technique into identical preeminent acupuncture procedures and applications, without having sufficient understanding and training of Acupuncture Physiology.

We, who are licensed in acupuncture and Oriental medicine, make this declaration to defend the 3000 + years of tradition which we cherish and honor.

I. Acupuncture Physiology[1] is Science.

Science simply defined is the observation of cause and effect in nature.

A. The secret of acupuncture's (and its related modalities) unquestionable success and efficacy is in the entirety of its structure. From clinical examination of pulse, tongue, auscultation, palpation, visual inspection, and SOAP intake questions; the diagnosis made on the information gathered; to the proper interventions. The entirety of scope has been what has made acupuncture so popular, with great acceptance amongst the public and by evidence of expanding usage of procedures within other medical settings.

B. We consider the components of Acupuncture Physiology to be applicable laws of science. Qi, The Five Elements, Yin/Yang are a remarkable melding of nature and logic, which emphasize balance and homeostasis. Systematic, observable, able to be manipulated and intervened upon, they are an extraordinary engineering construct of nature and man.

C. From the 'discovery' of malaria treatment to location of bitter receptors[iv] upon the heart, Western Science is only now beginning to discover what has been known and studied in Acupuncture and Oriental Medicine for centuries. It is an exciting time for both sciences as Western Medicine validates that of the East, and vice -versa[v].

---

1 Oriental Medicine is implied as part of the term "Acupuncture Physiology"

Acupuncture is certainly an innovative evolving medicine. Modern techniques (such as dry needling), methods, and co-interventions with western procedures are emerging across the globe. We promote the advancement of acupuncture procedures and techniques, but recognize the fundamental nature of Acupuncture Physiology beneath.

3,000 years of Acupuncture Physiology has earned its Right to be respected as science, with its language to be considered as preeminent.

II. Preeminence of the Language of Acupuncture

The language of Acupuncture and Oriental Medicine should be considered pre-eminent. We strongly oppose the "re-invention" of acupuncture terms and modalities.

A. Two examples of appropriating Acupuncture and its modalities, and re-branding them are...

1. Gua Sha[vi] has taken on the term of Graston Technique[vii] by Physical Therapist.
2. Dry Needle. As it expands beyond its appropriate scope, dry needle is being used to justify cosmetic[viii] acupuncture. Now incorporating the use of distal points, retention of needles, and electro stimulation, dry needle is everyday becoming identical to preeminent acupuncture techniques and procedures.

III. Inappropriate Expansion of Dry Needle Technique into Identical Acupuncture Procedures for other Applications.

A. The dry needle technique is used for musculo skeletal pain disorders. One of its main endeavors is to achieve a muscle "twitch" response or fasciculation, which re-balances muscle tone and alignment across joints for pain relief and structural improvement. Dry Needle requires a repeated thrust and pull technique, without retention of the needle. Due to the repeated thrust and pull into sensitive trigger point areas, dry needle is one of the most painful techniques utilizing an acupuncture needle.[ix] In the hands of an inexperienced practitioner dry needle is even more painful. In such cases the discomfort suffered by a patient may turn them off from seeking acupuncture in any form altogether.

B. We see the expansion of dry needle in procedure and application move beyond its original intended purpose.

Retention of needle, attachment of electrical stimulation, and distal point needling are examples of dry needle expansion beyond its original technique and away from its original intended application which was to stimulate muscle fasciculation. The expansion of dry needle is in reality, simply using identical procedures preeminently determined by acupuncture.

We have seen the expansion of dry needle in application.

Example #1 is that of Cosmetic Acupuncture, which some Physical Therapist are venturing into vis a vis with "dry needle"[x]. Based upon the discomfort of technique and application only for pain, it is completely inappropriate to categorize dry needle technique for facial cosmetic purposes.

Example #2 is the expanded use of dry needle technique into sinusitis conditions. With questionable training, dry needlers are now positioning themselves as sinusitis experts, although they likely have no understanding of the conditions leading to sinusitis, nor how to check pulse and tongue in diagnosing sinusitis. By the way, what kind of muscle twitch do you try to get when treating sinusitis with dry needle? Ouch!

Based upon the above example there leaves little doubt that the expansion of dry needle technique will be used as justification for out of scope non myofascial pain complaints.

IV. Use of identical acupuncture procedures in ignorance of Acupuncture Physiology.

A. The expansion of dry needle into other identical and preeminent acupuncture procedures for non myofascial pain applications puts both the practitioner and patient in the situation of being ignorant of said procedures and application.

Acupuncture's success is directly related to knowledge and understanding the science of Acupuncture Physiology, examination, diagnosis, and proper intervention.
In the cosmetic example above it is a mistake to consider the face in isolation to the entirety of structure. The face is a reflection of the entire body condition, physical, emotional, and psycho - spiritual, especially in regards to digestive, bowel function, general stress and fatigue.
In complete understanding of Acupuncture Physiology the licensed acupuncturist performs cosmetic acupuncture, considering the unique patterns presented by every individual. It is the same way for any application and intervention of acupuncture.

B. We believe Physical Therapists and others are trying to set a precedent for using dry needle and appropriated procedures as justification for expansion into other scopes of practice. Without proper understanding of Acupuncture Physiology we believe this to be unethical, misleading, and dangerous practice to the public.

V. Physical Therapy's own math indicates insufficient training of dry needle technique.

A. According to North Carolina's Physical Therapy Board lawsuit against North Carolina's Board of Acupuncture (Case No. 1:15-cv-831), Line item 35 states the following "According to a recent study by the Human Resources Research Organization, more than four-fifths (86%) of what physical therapists need to know to be competent in dry needling is acquired during the course of their clinical education alone. This includes knowledge related to evaluation, assessment, diagnosis and plan of care development, documentation, safety, and professional responsibilities."[xi]

In other words, a Physical Therapist still needs to have 14% additional clinical education hours of training to be sufficient in the practice of Dry Needle technique.

B. According to CAPTE Commission on Accreditation in Physical Therapy Education's Aggregate Program Data 2014 -2015 Physical Therapist Education Program Fact Sheets[xii]. Table 9 states the Mean Number of contact / clock hours in full time clinical education to be 1,421 hours.

C. Let's do the math. CAPTE's mean clinical education hours are 1,421. An additional 14% of clinical education is required for learning the dry needle technique. Therefore a Physical Therapist needs 198 hours (14% of 1421 hours) additional clinical training to be able to practice Dry Needle Technique.

Clinical hours do not exist in a vacuum. Behind them exists the didactic course and curriculum, which according to The CAPTE Aggregate Program Data 2014 -2015 Fact Sheet Figure 4 there is approximately 79.6 % of didactic / lab work in proportion to 20.4 % clinical education.
Therefore additional didactic study for the dry needle technique would require an almost additional 800 hours to the 198 hours of clinical dry needle training.

VI. Current Educational Requirements for a Physical Therapist to practice Dry Needle Technique.

In general (with variance amongst states), for a Physical Therapist to practice the dry needle technique 27-46 hours training are required in the use of needles. With a portion of those hours allowed to be home / online study[xiii].

VII. The conclusion according to Physical Therapist own math and clinical education is that 27 - 46 hours of education is grossly insufficient to be able to practice the dry needle technique.

    A. Furthermore the quality of these educational programs is questionable at best. There is one account of a class being provided with excellent didactic education, but when it came to the portion of hands on clinical education, chaos ensued as students fumbled with the most basic of skills like opening a pack of needles and within 20 minutes were dangerously inserting needles unsupervised. [xiv]

B. We see classes generally being taught in a "weekend warrior" type of environment where there can be as many as 60 or more students per one instructor[xv]. Physical therapist are then sent "home" after a weekend class to practice their clinical dry needle in an unsupervised environment[xvi]. These practices are a mockery of a true and proper clinical experience.

C. We believe current allowable training practices of dry needle by Physical Therapist to be thoroughly insufficient and inappropriate for learning an invasive medical procedure. We believe such training environments need to be investigated and regulated more closely.

VIII. Sections V through VII indicate only the training necessary to perform dry needle alone.

It is not accountable for the expansion of dry needle technique into identical pre existing, preeminent acupuncture techniques. The educational requirements met for the Dry Needlist to practice beyond dry needle falls close to 0% in knowledge of Acupuncture Physiology, distal point acupuncture and applications beyond pain.

IX. In Conclusion

We understand other profession's desire to want to incorporate our procedures into their own practices. The fact of the appropriation of our techniques is first evidence of their efficacy.
For purpose of safety and full disclosure to the public and patients we ask that anybody who wants to be able to practice acupuncture and oriental medicine to be properly and fully educated under a complete acupuncture and oriental medicine accredited training program.
We the authors thank you for your consideration of such matters.

i http://www.kinetacore.com/physical-therapy/Physical-Therapy-Training/page149.html

ii http://integrativedryneedling.com/resources/state-training-guidelines/

iii https://en.wikipedia.org/wiki/Dunning%E2%80%93Kruger_effect

iv https://www.uq.edu.au/news/article/2015/05/not-sweet-heart-researchers-find-bitter-taste-receptors-human-hearts, Walter Thomas. This corresponds to the classifications of taste to organs in Oriental Medicine. In classifying herbs the heart generally has an affinity for bitter taste.

v Acupuncture adjusts calcium levels to protect the body from ischemia (http://www.ncbi.nlm.nih.gov/m/pubmed/12584796/.
Acupuncture affects the nervous system to help it heal (https://www.hss.edu/.../Acupuncture-and-Neurophysiology.pdf).
Acupuncture allows the mind to relax into delta or theta states which decrease anxiety (http://www.ncbi.nlm.nih.gov/m/pubmed/23885609/).

vi https://en.wikipedia.org/wiki/Gua_sha

vii http://www.grastontechnique.com/

viii from a website promoting Cosmetic Dry Needling Using language the same as acupuncture.

ix http://www.everydayhealth.com/columns/my-health-story/dry-needling-most-painful-thing-ever-loved/

x ibid

xi Analysis of Competencies for Dry Needling by Physical Therapists, Joseph Caramagno Leslie Adrian Lorin Mueller Justin Purl, July 10,2015 page 13

xii http://www.capteonline.org/uploadedFiles/CAPTEorg/About_CAPTE/Resources/Aggregate_Program_Data/AggregateProgramData_PTPrograms.pdf

xiii http://www.keepacupuncturereal.com/

xiv http://www.liveoakacupuncture.com/dry-needling - "My experience at the "Dry Needling Certification" Course

xv ibid

xvixvixvixvi http://www.kinetacore.com/physical-therapy/Trigger-Point-Dry-Needling-Level-II-Training/page18.html

Violations of Acupuncture's Unified Competency Model

Acupuncture's unified competency model is a complete medical system explaining the human condition. Acupuncture's unified competency model entails the established language, procedures, acupuncture point locations and energetics, acupuncture and oriental medicine physiology, herbal medicine, examination procedures, diagnosis, assessment, treatment plan, and prognosis as taught in universities and in general clinical use worldwide. The unified competency model provides a basis for understanding and study of acupuncture and its related modalities and procedures amongst acupuncturist worldwide and across medical professions and sciences.[xvi]

Acupuncture's unified competency model has been established through educational institutions, journals, historical records, clinical standards of care, and the long traditions spanning the course of millennia. The classification of points, point locations, organization of points along channels to specific organs has long been established. As has been classification of diseases and pathologies such as wind, dry, damp, heat, cold, interior/ exterior disease, deficiency, excess, yin/ yang. Acupuncture's unified competency model seamlessly intertwines acupuncture point energetic and acupuncture intervention according to diagnosed patterns and pathologies exhibited in the patient.

Acupuncture's unified competency model does allow for new techniques and new understanding of the physiological effects measured in western models.

We acupuncturist, licensed in Acupuncture and Oriental Medicine, oppose attempts by therapeutic professionals utilizing dry needle technique to redefine and circumvent acupuncture's unified competency model, for purposes of their abbreviated training models. They do so by re-defining acupuncture's preeminent point energetics with general non specific language such as "homeostatic point and effect". They do so by re- naming the established nomenclature of acupuncture point locations. They do so as a means to avoid additional training needed to learn acupuncture and acupuncture physiology.

The use of this "homeostatic, neurologic language" has been justified by dry needle practitioners who reference Dr. Chan Gunn, Dr. Houchi Dung, and Dr. Yu Tan Ma. Dr. Dung and Dr. Ma were originally comprehensively trained acupuncturist, while Dr. Gunn states that his "IMS (technique) borrows its needle technique from traditional Chinese acupuncture."[xvi] Preeminent acupuncture points and procedures are the foundation from which dry needle branched from.

It has already been pointed out in "Arguments for the Defense of Acupuncture" section III and IV how dry needle practitioners are trying to expand the scope of dry needle technique to more than just the treatment of myofascial pain. The cosmetic procedure was used as an example of expansion of dry needle technique into preeminent acupuncture procedures. Since then dry needle for sinus relief has reared itself up as well.

It was pointed out how the scope of dry needle technique is being expanded to the use of distal related acupuncture points and needle retention. Dry needle technique is a branch from the foundations of acupuncture. As dry needle practitioners try to expand the scope of dry needle they are simply returning to the foundation of preeminent principles and procedures of acupuncture, albeit without proper understanding.

This is where dry needle practitioners are violating acupuncture's competency model. They are redefining acupuncture energetic point functions in language such as "homeostatic, neurologic effect". Using such language serves as justification in the mind of a dry needle practitioner to perform acupuncture (and all that it can treat) in the absence of knowledge of acupuncture physiology.
Such was the case in a public post on facebook by an Ohio physical therapist for using acupuncture point HeGu, Large Intestine 4 for the treatment of a headache. "Dry needling the homeostatic point of the superficial radial nerve for headaches and migraines works!" they posted with a picture on December 23rd, 2015.

First off this is another clear example of the inappropriate expansion of dry needle, beyond myofascial effect. It is simply the use of a preeminent distal acupuncture point with needle retention and has nothing to do with musculoskeletal pain (as dry needle was originally intended for). As wonderful as the physical therapist in Ohio makes Large Intestine 4 sound for the treatment of headaches, their comment demonstrates their vast ignorance of acupuncture physiology behind the use of Large Intestine 4. There is no differentiation of headache according to location, frequency, severity, and accompanying symptoms. There is no proper diagnosis for the cause of the headache. They simply promote L.I. 4 as a panacea for all types of headaches, which is inappropriate and demonstrates an incomplete understanding of headaches and an ignorance of acupuncture physiology behind the cause of headaches.

We do not have a problem with modern science validating the function of acupuncture. It certainly has been confirmed that acupuncture does cause homeostatic, neurologic changes and effects to the endocrine system involving hypothalamus, adrenals/ thyroid and pituitary glands. Just because the effects of acupuncture are being validated by western science should not allow a western trained therapeutic practitioner to use acupuncture without an appropriate background in acupuncture physiology. Effecting neurologic homeostatic change is not justification for practicing acupuncture.
Due to the desire to circumvent the burden of additional training in acupuncture and oriental medicine, dry needle practitioners are forced in the awkward position of having to disregard the preeminence of the acupuncture procedures they perform. Even in the study of dry needle technique they do not have sufficient training (section V of "Arguments for the Defense of Acupuncture). This is a core problem of physical therapist practicing dry needle today. Often they boast of extensive training and knowledge in anatomy (which is great) but when it comes to understanding physiology and the energetics of acupuncture, they know nothing. Even though in some cases, the core of their practice and livelihood is the use of preeminent acupuncture procedures.

As stated in Arguments for the Defense of Acupuncture, "the expansion of dry needle into other identical and preeminent acupuncture procedures for non myofascial pain applications puts both the practitioner and patient in the situation of being ignorant of said procedures and application." It is simply unethical and malpractice for a practitioner to be performing a technique for which they nor the patient have no understanding of the underlying physiology.

If the dry needle practitioner were to regard acupuncture as the basis of their procedures they would have to admit themselves to the time and training of learning it. In order to avoid this they have turned to violating acupuncture's unified competency model by renaming acupuncture points and functions.

On page 216 of Yu Tan Ma's book "Biomedical Acupuncture for Pain Management" he teaches point locations for asthma and sinusitis, naming the points HAs, PAs, and SAs. Dr. Dung is referenced by the Ohio physical therapist in justifying L.I. 4 as a homeostatic effect. These doctors originally and comprehensively trained in acupuncture are no authorities in allowing the language of acupuncture to change, particularly doing so to suit the needs of their customers who want to circumvent proper education.

Acupuncture physiology does not change. Acupuncture physiology and the insertion of a needle are intertwined. They complement one another. Developed over thousands of years they are a complete system for understanding and treating illness. Dry needle is in its infancy[xvi] (as stated by physical therapist) and is dwarfed by the complete system of acupuncture and oriental medicine. Dry needle practitioners do not have the right to re-define the preeminent procedures, point locations, functions, in order to suit their need of having an abbreviated education.

When a needle is inserted, it affects acupuncture physiology. Inserting needles without a diagnosis, or understanding of acupuncture physiology is unethical and malpractice as both the patient and practitioner are ignorant of principles of preeminent acupuncture being used.

Acupuncture has established its unified competency model and preeminence based upon traditions and cumulative experiences over thousands of years. The unified competency model allows acupuncturist to clearly exchange ideas with one another and across medical professions and sciences without confusion. It allows acupuncturist to study historical records and journals without confusion. Acupuncture's unified competency model allows the profession to grow and improve.

Acupuncture's competency model allows dry needle, or muscle trigger point to be a branch of it, which is the correct place for dry needle. Dry needle is a branch. Dry needle is not the distal retention of needles; it is not for conditions other than myofascial pain. Expanding the use of dry needle into other applications is simply the use of preeminent acupuncture procedures, for which the roots of application have been established in acupuncture's unified competency model.

For those wishing to add acupuncture to their practice, learn it completely at an accredited acupuncture institution.

xvi https://c.ymcdn.com/sites/www.aaaomonline.org/resource/resmgr/Committees-Education/Acupuncture_Competency_Model.pdf. AAAOMonline.org/? competencies
xvi http://www.istop.org/drgunn.html
xvi xvi http://www.apta.org/PTinMotion/2015/5/DryNeedling/

My comment to an article by Kristen Horner Warren "What you must know before you try dry needling". *

From her article in a dry needle class for physical therapist. The whole experience made me think of the Dunning-Kruger Effect. According to the Journal of Personality and Social Psychology:
The Dunning–Kruger effect is a cognitive bias wherein unskilled individuals suffer from illusory superiority, mistakenly assessing their ability to be much higher than is accurate. This bias is attributed to a metacognitive inability of the unskilled to recognize their ineptitude. Conversely, highly skilled individuals tend to underestimate their relative competence, erroneously assuming that tasks which are easy for them are also easy for others.

My comment on her article.

I experienced firsthand the Dunning–Kruger when I was patient in the hands of a chiropractor who also practiced "acupuncture". I was a patient ignorant of how acupuncture worked. Being ignorant, I fully trusted that the chiropractor was qualified, skilled, and experienced to practice acupuncture. Unfortunately he was not. I thought it a little strange when he was saying to himself "let's see heart problems, heart problems" as he thumbed through a book at his side. "Ah yes, here it is." he said and proceeded to needle me with two points in the area of the thumb. That is all he did as I sat there for about 15 minutes with the needles in my thumbs. He performed no consultation, no examination, and no diagnoses of my condition. Afterwards he sent me home with some expensive bottle of extract he recommended.

Needless to say his 'acupuncture' didn't work. I was discouraged and believed acupuncture didn't work for me. As my condition turned more severe and I was on the brink of death, in desperation I again sought out an acupuncturist. This time I found a real qualified acupuncturist who properly understood my condition, performed and examination, gave me an explanation and diagnosis of my disease, and treated my condition accordingly. It is what saved my life and what got me interested in learning more about acupuncture.

Seeing a real qualified acupuncturist is what provided for me a most miraculous healing experience and adventure that continues to this day, 14 years later. I am now a doctor of acupuncture and oriental medicine. As I remember my experience as a patient, when I was ignorant and went to see that chiropractor, I have nothing but contempt and anger for the "system" which allowed him to practice a medical procedure upon me for which he had no proper training and understanding of. I was the victim of unethical medical malpractice.

I know the points he used on me, they were Large intestine 4 bi laterally. These are very commonly used acupuncture, acupressure points. They are good for many things, but utterly inappropriate for the heart condition I was suffering from. I want to warn the public about my experience. Unfortunately it is getting worse and becoming more common as overzealous dry needle practitioners suffering from the Dunning–Kruger effect, perform dry needle beyond their capabilities. Thank god I found a real qualified acupuncturist who truly understood my condition. It began the greatest, most wonderful miracle of my life. Please, please make sure you inquire into the training and experience of those who are putting needles into you. They may have no experience and no understanding of the medicine they claim to be practicing.

* http://www.liveoakacupuncture.com/before-you-try-dry-needling

Concerns and cautions regarding the practice of Dry Needle technique by non acupuncturist.
Patient warning: Don't be a Guinea Pig for your dry needle practitioner in training.

Many professionals in the health care community are shocked and highly concerned regarding the current practices by Physical Therapists and their boards in allowing the practice of Dry Needling with insufficient training. The American Academy of Medical Acupuncturist (an association of 1,200 medical doctors with training in acupuncture) have published multiple papers warning the public about public health and safety issues regarding practice of dry needling by physical therapist.

From the AAMA "Policy on Dry Needling" statement "Physical therapy is not a field that has historically included the use of needles. The recent trend of some physical therapists to embrace dry needling under the umbrella of physical therapy practice is one that marks a distinct departure from traditional physical therapy practice. The fact that many physical therapists receive only minimal hours of training speaks to the potential danger of their practice….Therefore, the AAMA strongly believes that, for the health and safety of the public, this procedure should be performed only by practitioners with extensive training and familiarity with routine use of needles in their practice and who are duly licensed to perform these procedures, such as licensed medical physicians or licensed acupuncturists. In our experience and medical opinion, it is inadvisable legally to expand the scope of physical therapists to include dry needling as part of their practice."

Why the concern of Medical Doctors and Acupuncture Professionals? Even by the standards set by Physical Therapists themselves[xvi] they are practicing dry needle on an unsuspecting public with insufficient training. [xvi] According to papers written by the Commission on Accreditation in Physical Therapy 2014 -2015 Fact Sheet and "Analysis of Competencies for Dry Needling by Physical Therapist" the minimum hours of training before allowing a Physical Therapist to practice dry needle should be at least 400 hours, which should take place in a proper and well supervised clinical setting.

Unfortunately current practices by Physical Therapist fall far short of their own measures. In most states only between 24 -50 hours in education are needed for a Physical Therapist to practice dry needle upon the public. These training programs are often a mockery of a proper clinical setting; taken in weekend warrior settings, with too few staff and too many students. Worse yet, physical therapist are sent home after the weekend with instructions to practice upon their patients in order to fulfill their clinical education requirements. The patient is the guinea pig for which the Dry Needle practitioner is expected to hone their technique.

xvi
http://www.capteonline.org/uploadedFiles/CAPTEorg/About_CAPTE/Resources/Aggregate_Program_Data/AggregateProgramData_PTPrograms.pdf
xvi xvi Analysis of Competencies for Dry Needling by Physical Therapists, Joseph Caramagno Leslie Adrian Lorin Mueller Justin Purl, July 10,2015 page 13

**Controversy and unethical practices surrounding dry needle technique.
What every patient should know.**

The controversy surrounding dry needling is not limited to whether physical therapist or other non acupuncture therapist should be sticking needles in patients without sufficient training. It extends to the slippery slope of dry needle technique expansion into preeminent acupuncture procedures and protocols without the underlying understanding of acupuncture physiology.

The dry needle technique is used for musculo skeletal pain disorders. One of its main endeavors is to achieve a muscle "twitch" response or fasciculation, which re-balances muscle tone and alignment across joints for pain relief and structural improvement. Dry Needle requires a repeated thrust and pull technique, without retention of the needle.[xvi]

Unfortunately numerous examples abound of dry needle practitioners expanding the scope of dry needling into retention of needle, attachment of electrical stimulation, and distal point needling away from its original application which was to stimulate muscle fasciculation. The expansion of dry needle is in reality, simply using identical procedures preeminently determined by acupuncture.[xvi] This speaks to the limitation of the dry needle technique itself. In the hands of a qualified practitioner dry needle can achieve good results. In the hands of a poorly skilled practitioner it can cause harm. Dry needling is not a 'cure all'. If it was then the addition of distal acupuncture points, retention of needle, and other preeminent acupuncture modalities would not be necessary.
The slippery slope, loophole used by dry needle practitioners is that all acupuncture procedures are now simply being rebranded as dry needling. By doing so the dry needle practitioner can practice acupuncture without training, nor understanding of acupuncture physiology underlying the acupuncture they practice.

The expansion of dry needling into the use of acupuncture by physical therapist and other non acupuncture therapist speaks to the superior efficacy acupuncture and its preeminent modalities and procedures as therapy. There may be no greater proof than others simply trying to copy acupuncture's procedures.

Unfortunately acupuncture is a victim of its own success. The youth and small size of the acupuncture profession in the United States makes it difficult to speak truth to the public about what is happening to its medicine. Acupuncturist are concerned for their careers and for the correct, ethical, righteous practice of acupuncture and its preeminent modalities.

With the proliferation of dry needling, quality and ethical standards will decline. The public will be misled as dry needling expands its scope beyond the treatment of myofascial pain complaints. Both the dry needle practitioner and patient will be ignorant of the acupuncture physiology beneath the acupuncture techniques they are practicing.

Acupuncture will be practiced without proper examination, assessment, diagnosis, and prognosis. Seamlessly intertwined with acupuncture physiology are 3000 years of acupuncture, its preeminent procedures and modalities, and the extraordinary engineering human construct of oriental medicine. The public will be fooled into believing their dry needle therapist with under 50 hours in training has even an inkling of understanding into such things.

xvi "Arguments for the Defense of Acupuncture" Evan Mahoney, undisclosed co - authors, expected publication FSOMA journal 2016

xvi ibid

A Needle Phobic Acupuncturist

I am an Acupuncturist. I have had over 3000 hours of training in Acupuncture and Oriental Medicine from properly accredited acupuncture schools. This included hundreds of treatments in clinical training under proper supervision of my school teachers who were experts in acupuncture and needling therapies. This does not include the hours spent in the classroom learning and practicing over 360 acupuncture points, their precise location, needle insertion techniques, depth, safety, and contraindications of the acupuncture points.

I am pleased to have been so well trained and versed in this great medicine. With 3000 + years of history it is great to be a part of its movement into the west. Acupuncture is turning heads everywhere and winning over skeptics patient by patient. Acupuncture is certainly recognized as effective for a multitude of illnesses and pain diseases.

Unfortunately though, acupuncture is also becoming a victim of its own success. The heads turning towards acupuncture are not just skeptical patients, but others in the health care profession who wish to appropriate acupuncture as their own, with only the most minimal and negligible training standards in place. This is the source of my needle phobia.

Like phobias of spiders, snakes, and heights, needle phobia may be at the top of the list for some members of the public. It may be the biggest obstacle in bringing more people to acupuncture. I have had many patients speak to me of their fear of needles, prior to receiving their first ever acupuncture treatment. Because of my skill, training, and experience in acupuncture and oriental medicine I am able to confidently assure them of their utmost comfort. Because of my extensive training in acupuncture I have a multitude of techniques at hand for which to suit my patient's needs.

I have great dexterity and skill in my needle handling and technique. This is borne from the stages of learning acupuncture to practicing acupuncture. The stages which begin in ignorance with exuberance and overzealousness, through experience become something akin to fear and reticence.

"Acupuncture is easy to learn, difficult to practice" is something I picked up somewhere in one of my text books, or maybe said by a teacher. It is easy to become exuberant when learning acupuncture; it is easy to internalize this medicine and its theories. It is easy to witness the gears of this great human engineering construct as one heals themselves (as most students do) and then heals others.

Born from experience and seasoned maturity is the realization of responsibility the acupuncturist holds for their patients, of providing honest ethical guidance while at the same time delivering results. This includes knowledge of the complexity of human illness and pain and the uniqueness of every patient. This is the difficulty of practicing acupuncture. This is where the years and thousands of hours of training make the difference. This is why I have no fear of submitting myself for a treatment from a properly licensed acupuncturist, educated in a properly accredited acupuncture school.

This is also why I share my needle phobia with members of the general public. Behind the scenes and veiled from the public I see the current practices going on by other health care practitioners who are trying to incorporate the success of acupuncture into their own fields. I am fearful of these practices.

With as little as 27 to 50 hours of education, which includes both didactic and minimal unregulated clinical practice, typically occurring in the course of a weekend or two, the dry needle practitioner is sent home able to stick needles in their patients.

To put it into context, the training necessary for these practitioners is the equivalent of half a semester of an acupuncturist in their first quarter of school, which corresponds to the exuberant, overzealous phase of one's acupuncture education.

It is a horrifying prospect to imagine being a patient and lying face down on the table while somebody with inadequate training begins to finger and palpate the muscles of my neck, prepping for needle insertion. This is the dry needle technique. This is this technique which allows someone with only 27 to 50 hours to insert needles into patients.

I know and practice dry needle technique myself. It is the most painful and aggressive acupuncture technique performed. It requires the practitioner to deeply and repeatedly push and pull the needle with the intent of eliciting a "muscle twitch" response. I also know the limits of the dry needle technique. A muscle twitch is not always elicited. I know when to stop and when to incorporate other acupuncture techniques. This is the difference of 3000 + hours of acupuncture education. Fear and reticence are attributes born from the long experience of education and practice.

The 27-50 hour dry needle therapist does not have this caution born of experience. They are prone to over exuberance, overzealousness documented by the Dunning -Kruger Effect.

The Dunning–Kruger effect is a cognitive bias wherein unskilled individuals suffer from illusory superiority, mistakenly assessing their ability to be much higher than is accurate. This bias is attributed to a metacognitive inability of the unskilled to recognize their ineptitude. Conversely, highly skilled individuals tend to underestimate their relative competence, erroneously assuming that tasks which are easy for them are also easy for others (Wikipedia).

Worse yet, as an acupuncturist, I see how the limitations of the dry needle technique lead the unskilled practitioner turn to more traditional acupuncture. They begin to retain their needles and use traditional acupuncture point locations, or distal acupuncture location. Suddenly they are using more needles. Blindly and in ignorance they think they can simply practice acupuncture without training and knowledge of its principles.

Now, not only is it horrifying, but it is maddening. Both the patient and practitioner are ignorantly engaged in acupuncture. This should not have been allowed to happen. I am fearful for the patient lying prone on the table in the hands of someone with so little experience in acupuncture and needle therapy. For one who is needle phobic, it is a nightmare scenario.

The Judgment is Severe

It should be known, in the views of some in the acupuncture profession.

Acupuncture is supercedant and antecedent to dry needle. Acupuncture's influence is broad and numerous, with unfolding branches unto today.

I-Ching, Dynastys, Yellow Emperor, Kings and Doctors, Korea, Japan. Yin/Yang, The Five Elements, Qi, Biomedical Acupuncture, Muscle Releasing Acupuncture, TaiChi, Qi Gong, Meditation. The Schools of Moxa, The schools of Heat and Cold. The understanding of examination, diagnosis, and prognosis based upon the precepts of oriental medicine and science.

The ability to act ethically as a practitioner.

These numerous applications existent for ions, are yet in their infancy of broadening human understanding, nature, spirit, encompassing all health and disease. Like a living organism still evolving through sentient experience and accumulated knowledge. An octopus of exploration and discovery lies ahead.

Through Acupuncture and Oriental Medicine the libraries of Alexandria shall be built again. Western philosophies and religions will be reconciled to new truths.

Let it be known that Acupuncture antedates, dry needle. Dry Needle, is a subset in the broad canon of acupuncture.

Used for argument and influence: Anyone who puts forth the opposing position that dry needle somehow supersedes acupuncture, that acupuncture is only a subset of dry needle.

The Judgment is severe. Anyone so ignorant, who holds such views, should be prohibited from practicing needle therapy.

To counter such ignorance, Acupuncture and Oriental Medicine needs to be incorporated with today's public and private education. Through being placed in said institutions that teach a broad array of arts, humanities, and sciences.

There is a growing demand and need for educational diversity. Acupuncture and Oriental Medicine has demonstrated the validity, truth, and wisdom, applied through the ages both in the subjective and objective senses.

Acupuncture's Dry Needle Technique /Muscle Trigger Point therapy xvi

Following are eight mechanisms involving the pathology of muscle trigger points. An acupuncturist uses various techniques from which to address the mechanisms of muscle trigger point pathology including the dry needle acupuncture, which is often seamlessly intertwined with traditional acupuncture and other pre-eminent techniques of acupuncture and oriental medicine.

Trigger points are knots or nodules located in muscle tissue. The first mechanism that occurs due to the presence of knots in the muscle tissue is that the muscle becomes "SHORTENED". The analogy is if you take a piece of rope and tie it into a knot, it will shorten the length of that rope. Knots (Trigger Points) are clusters of fascia which tangle up and shorten the length of muscle.

The second mechanism that occurs due to trigger points is that they add increased tension and strain on the tendons. If the muscle is shortened it adds more strain on the tendon. A stretched and tightened tendon will likely rub with increased friction against adjacent tissues. Tendinitis (inflammation of the tendon) and muscle strains/ sprains are the most common injuries and diagnosis resulting from shortened muscles.

The third mechanism that occurs due to the presence of trigger points is the range of motion of the joint or limb will be decreased. The pull and strain from the shortened muscle and tightened tendon, simply will not allow the full range of motion of the joint or limb. When we do accidentally twist our foot or limb beyond its inhibited range of motion, a muscle sprain or strain will occur. Further damage such as a tear can also occur.

Fourth mechanism that occurs due to the presence of trigger points is that they inhibit the circulation of blood and oxygen to the muscle tissue. Blood and oxygen have a harder time circulating through the cluster of knotted tissue and fascia. The muscle becomes dehydrated. Dr. Hyungsuk Choi of Samra Acupuncture Center states the muscle tissue becomes a "Beef Jerky" like consistency, very dry and stringy. xvi

Fifth Mechanism, a muscle that is dry and stringy with trigger points is unable to be strengthened. To strengthen, you must restore it to its normal length, tenderness, and pliability first.

Sixth Mechanism, the trigger point is painful upon palpation. The pain felt does not have to be local to the trigger point area. Pain will refer to points where the muscle attaches and inserts. Many painful diseases are actually located distantly away from where the trigger point occurs.

Seventh Mechanism is that trigger points can be present without any pain or physical complaint. Until a triggering event occurs (like accident, injury, or exposure to cold and ice). There may be no physical complaint even though the trigger point is present.

Eighth Mechanism: Peripheral Nerve Impingement. A shortened muscle/ stretched tendon may pinch on the nerves at the periphery (outside of the spinal column) causing radiating pain, numbness, or tingling down arms or joints. This is a more favorable prognosis as muscle stretching / tendon relaxation will eliminate the nerve impingement.

Acupuncture's Dry Needle / Muscle Trigger Point therapy is an excellent way to get pain relief and return to full activity.

xvi Excerpts taken from "Saam Korean Acupuncture: Advanced Combinations" copyright 2013 by Evan Mahoney
xvi Choi, Hyungsuk, Hamsoa Childrens Hospital, Los Angeles, Korea. This quote was taught to me verbally by Dr. Choi during my training under him at Samra Acupuncture Center.

Acupuncture's Dry Needle Technique /Muscle Trigger Point Therapy

Agonist/ Antagonist Muscle identification.

In Acupuncture's Dry Needle Technique/ Muscle Trigger Point Therapy the acupuncturist can identify the antagonist muscle in need of treatment through range of motion examination. If there is limitation in range of motion, the antagonist muscle is identified as the muscle prohibiting the full range of motion of joint or limb.

Agonist Muscle: Muscle that initiates the action of movement of limb or body part.

Antagonist Muscle: Muscle that counters the action of agonist muscle, and creates movement of limb or body part counter to that of the agonist. The antagonist is identified as the shortened muscle causing the decrease in range of motion, of joint or limb.i

An example of the agonist / antagonist muscle is the biceps and triceps in flexion and extension of the forearm. To flex the forearm the biceps muscle initiates the movement. The biceps muscle contracts to move the forearm, it is the agonist muscle. While the biceps is contracting, the triceps extends and relaxes to allow the full movement of the joint or limb. The triceps muscle is the antagonist muscle when the forearm is flexing.

To extend the forearm the triceps muscle initiates the movement. The triceps contracts to straighten the forearm, it is the agonist muscle. As the forearm straightens, the biceps muscle extends and relaxes to allow the full movement. The biceps muscle is the antagonist muscle when the forearm extends. In the previous article outlining the eight mechanisms of muscle trigger point pathology, the first mechanism of the presence of knots in a muscle is that the muscle becomes shortened. In the antagonist role a muscle that is shortened will not allow for the full movement of joint or limb. In the above example if the triceps muscle is shortened due to the presence of knots, the full extension of the forearm will be limited. The patient will not be able to fully straighten their arm.

An acupuncturist will have at their disposal the ability to perform dry needle acupuncture upon the triceps muscle. With the proper placement of the needle into the trigger point a twitch response may be elicited. This twitch response is an involuntary contraction of the muscle that essentially shakes out or unties the knot in the muscle. Afterwards the muscle is elongated and relaxed. Tension upon the tendon which attaches the muscle to the bone is relaxed. This will allow for fuller extension of the muscle when in the antagonist role. Fuller range of motion will be achieved.

A word of caution, dry needle is not the 'cure all'. A properly trained and qualified acupuncturist has many tools at their disposal to achieve the benefits outlined above. Dry needle may be used in conjunction with these other therapies.

i Saam Korean Acupuncture: Advanced Combinations, Evan Mahoney, page 33, 2013

Acupuncture's Dry Needle and the Tensegrity Model

The Tensegrity Model was first coined by Buckminster Fuller in his explanation of spherical structures and forces maintaining stability of structures. "He explored these ideas through studies of the close-packing of spheres and tensile and compressive stabilization models, noting that tension and compression are not opposites, but rather complements that can be found together; when the two forces are harmonious, continuous pull is balanced by equally discontinuous pushing forces. This synergy between compression and tension is what Fuller calls tensegrity, "a system that stabilizes itself mechanically because of the way in which tensional and compressive forces are distributed and balanced within the structure (Ingber 48-9)". [1]

"On an anatomical level, the human body provides a good example of a prestressed tensegrity structure. Bones act as struts resisting the pull of tensile muscles, tendons and ligaments. Moreover, the stability of the shape of the body, or its stiffness, of the body is a function of the tone, or prestress, of its muscles (Ingber Lab). As Ingber puts it, "We are 206 compression-resistant bones that are pulled up against the force of gravity and stabilized through a connection with a continuous series of tensile tendons, muscles, and ligaments" (Ingber Lab)." [2]

Tensegrity and Muscle Shortening

Muscle shortening causes increased stress and pressure upon the tendons and supporting structures that are attached to the shortened muscle. Dr. Hyungsuk Choi in his explanation of Korean Kinetic Acupuncture implies that uneven muscle tension along the spine causes it to pull to the side of the shortened contracted muscles, which are exerting higher tension. "When we treat a patient's back pain, we do not work directly on the spine, but rather on the muscles attached to it. By using acupuncture, we can balance the tension of muscles and eventually obtain the proper stance of the spine." [3]
Like a chain reaction of events, an imbalance in one area can spread to other areas over the whole body. A patient with a history of ankle or foot injury could develop neck or TMJ problems as balance has shifted and the forces of tensegrity have rebalanced from the ankle, to the knees, hips, back, to the neck and shoulders.

Dr. Jonghwa Lee's VST (Vertex Synchronizing Technique) Acupuncture is a dry needle equivalent that measures range of motion imbalance along coronal, transverse, and sagittal plane analysis. "In such cases where tensegrity has shifted we will see evidence of imbalance, through difference in extremity length in the coronal plane analysis, pelvic and shoulder joint external and internal rotation differences in the transverse plane analysis, and curvature of the vertebra of the sagittal plane analysis. [4]

1. Verdier, Renee, "Animal Architecture: Buckminster Fuller's Tensegrity" Renee Verdier Blog. 3/2/09 www.realitysandwich.com/animal_architecture_buckminster_fuller_tensegrity
2. Verdier, Renee - ibid
3. Choi, Hyung Suk, Samra Acupuncture Center brochure page 6, published 2009 by Samra Acupuncture center
4. Lee, Jonghwa, Choi, Hyungsuk, Lee, Woongkyung Lee, Dongyup. "Vertex Synchronizing Technique Acupuncture (Tensegrity Model Acuppuncture) conference article 2009 Society for Acupuncture Research – Translational Research in Acupuncture: bridging Science, Practice and Community (SAR 2010), Chapel Hill, North Carolina March 19-21 2010

Acupuncture's Dry Needle Techinique - The Neck and Shoulder Vertex of VST Acupuncture (Vertex Synchronizing Technique)

VST acupuncture is a Dry Needle equivalent technique founded by Dr. Jonghwa Lee of Korea. It was taught as part of Samra University's DAOM program (now defunct) in Los Angeles, California. VST acupuncture uses range of motion analysis across transverse, coronal, and sagittal planes to identify antagonistic muscle restrictions. "VST acupuncture is relevantly designed with physical examination and its corresponding treatment. The main purpose is emphasized in balanced normalization of all connective tissue including the fascia and the muscle for maintaining tensegrity of the whole body. Tensegrity structures can be ruined by adhesions in muscle or fascia layers causing resistance in their sliding movement and by the tightness of muscles" [i]

Neck and Shoulder Vertex: Includes the muscles of the neck and shoulder which are tested for imbalances using range of motion tests and length measurements. The muscles of the neck and shoulder vertex for the purpose of this article are latismus dorsi, trapezius, infraspinatus, supraspinatus, teres minor, teres major, and levator scapulae.

Identification of Antagonist Muscles for Neck and Shoulder Pain in VST acupuncture.
For neck and shoulder pain patients we identify differences in tensegrity and the affected antagonist muscle through coronal plane analysis of measuring arm length differences and transverse plane analysis of internal rotation and external rotation of the shoulders. Through this analysis we will be able to target the affected muscle tissues.

If there is a difference in arm length at the coronal plane we thus identify it as the Latismus Dorsi and Teres Major muscles on the shortened side which are contracted and pulling the arm downward. In this case the Latismus Dorsi and Teres Major Muscles are the antagonist muscles.

For shoulder joint testing in the transverse plane, internal rotation restriction of the shoulder is correlated to the antagonist muscles Infraspinatus and Teres Minor of the affected side. For external rotation restriction of the shoulder the antagonists muscle is subscapularis.

Limitations of range of motion to the lateral rotation and bending of the head indicate restriction of the trapezius and levator scapulae muscles with possible involvement of the sternocleidomastoid and scalene muscles.

Per the analysis from coronal and transverse analysis we will have identified the affected antagonist muscles that are limiting the ROM. It is these muscles that are contracted and shortened and likely to have trigger points. We treat thus by using acupuncture and/or with dry needle to release the muscle trigger point.

[i] Lee, Jonghwa, Choi, Hyungsuk, Lee, Woongkyung Lee, Dongyup. "Vertex Synchronizing Technique Acupuncture (Tensegrity Model Acuppuncture, page 3-4 Conference article 2009 Society for Acupuncture Research – Translational Research in Acupuncture: bridging Science, Pracitice and Community (SAR 2010), Chapel Hill, North Carolina March 19-21 2010

Acupuncture's Dry Needle Technique - The Hip and Lower Back Vertex of VST Acupuncture (Vertex Synchronizing Technique)

Agonist/ Antagonist Muscles in VST

Every movement in the body has an agonist muscle (muscle initiating the action of movement) and an antagonist (muscle countering the action of movement). In VST acupuncture; which is a dry needle equivalent technique, we seek to identify and treat the antagonist muscle, which is the muscle that is shortened and is restricting the full range of motion of the limb or body part being moved.

Identification of Antagonist Muscles for Low Back Pain in VST

For lower back pain patients we identify differences in tensegrity and the affected antagonist muscle using coronal plane analysis of measuring leg length differences and transverse plane analysis of internal rotation of the hips. Through this analysis we will be able to target the affected muscle tissues. If there is a difference in leg length at the coronal plane we thus identify it as the Gluteus Maximus muscle on the shortened side is contracted and is pulling the pelvis downward [i] (barring any structural differences in limb length). In this case the Gluteus Maximus muscle is the antagonist preventing the hip from its normal range of motion.

In the coronal plane if we find restriction in lateral bending of the trunk then the identified antagonist muscle is the Quadratus Lumborum to the affected side. For hip joint testing in the transverse plane, internal rotation restriction of the hips is correlated to the antagonist muscles Tensor Fascia Latae (TFL) and Gluteus Medius, and Piriformis muscles of the affected side. For external rotation restriction the antagonists muscle are oblique abdominals, sartorious, and psoas.[ii]

Per the analysis from coronal and transverse analysis we will have identified the affected antagonist muscles that are limiting the ROM. It is these muscles that are contracted and shortened and likely to have trigger points. We treat thus by using acupuncture and/or with dry needle to release the muscle trigger point.

There are layers upon layers of thick muscle tissue in the lower back, so it is often difficult to generate a twitch response from dry needle upon the Gluteus muscles. Therefore in lieu of dry needle, acupuncture is usually performed with retention of needle upon the combined ashi / trigger point areas and the traditional acupuncture point locations of the lower back. This affords an example of a seamless interaction of dry needle and acupuncture.

Due to the limitations of the dry needle technique, preeminent traditional acupuncture point locations are also used. It is highly recommended to seek out a professionally trained and licensed acupuncturist who has the appropriate clinical and didactic training and knowledge to safely perform these techniques.

[i] Lee, Jonghwa, Choi, Hyungsuk, Lee, Woongkyung Lee, Dongyup. "Vertex Synchronizing Technique Acupuncture (Tensegrity Model Acuppuncture) conference article 2009 Society for Acupuncture Research – Translational Research in Acupuncture: bridging Science, Pracitice and Community (SAR 2010), Chapel Hill, North Carolina March 19-21 2010
[ii] Lee, Jonghwa "VST study guide from Samra University lecture" pages 2-3 2009

Limitations of the Dry Needle Technique

As mentioned in the joint article "VST Acupuncture Hip and Lower Back" the dry needle technique has its limitations. The first and primary limitation is that a muscle twitch response is not always elicited from the insertion of the needle. In this authors experience of practicing dry needle the only muscle that may regularly be predicted to have an elicited twitch response is the trapezius muscle of the neck. Perhaps it is due to the ability of the practitioner to easily palpate the muscle between the fingers as the patient lies prone (rendering it easy to find the trigger points) or if the trapezius is a muscle that simply carries more tension upon it. After the trapezius, getting a muscle twitch response is not assured and frequently rare.

This explains the phenomena of why dry needle practitioners without appropriate training and knowledge of acupuncture will use tens or even hundreds of needles tracing along the course of a muscle. The use of so many needles is an indication that they have failed to initiate a muscle twitch response.

The second limitation of the Dry Needle technique is that it is painful. Due to the repeated thrust and pull into sensitive trigger point areas of muscles, dry needle is one of the most painful techniques utilizing an acupuncture needle.[i] In the hands of a practitioner who over zealously searches for the twitch response dry needle is even more painful.[ii] Compounded with a general "needle phobia" amongst the public, dry needle in the hands of an inexperienced and inappropriately trained practitioner can simply be a nightmare for some patients to undergo. Licensed acupuncturist are very concerned for the comfort of patients during acupuncture and are concerned that the discomfort suffered from dry needle may turn patients away from acupuncture altogether.

Due to the limitations in eliciting a twitch response and effectiveness of the technique itself, dry needle often necessitates interaction with preeminent Traditional Acupuncture Techniques. This is where the retention of needle, use of distal points, use of electro - stimulation upon the needles, and other preeminent acupuncture techniques come into play. This is where the dry needle technique departs from being dry needle and where ethical issues of inappropriate and inadequately trained practitioners of acupuncture come into question.

A properly licensed and trained acupuncturist will have over two thousand hours of training in the field of acupuncture and oriental medicine, in a properly regulated clinical and didactic setting. Current practices of dry needle by non acupuncturist might as well be considered to be done in a "wild west" type atmosphere. Minimal training requirements in minimally regulated clinical and didactic settings by many dry needle practitioners are a huge cause of concern. For safety, comfort, and assurance that they are being treated by someone with complete knowledge of acupuncture, patients should always inquire into the credentials of their dry needle / acupuncture practitioner.

i http://www.everydayhealth.com/columns/my-health-story/dry-needling-most-painful-thing-ever-loved/
ii "Arguments for the Defense of Acupuncture and its Related Modalities and Procedures", expected publication 2016, FSOMA journal

What many in the Acupuncture Profession want you to know about the Dry Needle Technique.

The Dry Needle Technique is performed to achieve pain relief from musculoskeletal imbalance due to the muscle shortening effect of trigger points located within the fascia of the muscle tissue. The dry needle technique involves the insertion and probing of a needle to elicit a "muscle twitch" response which serves to relax and lengthen the muscle, thereby restoring balance and reduction in pain. In true practice the needle is not retained during the Dry Needle Technique.

The Limitations of the Dry Needle Technique.

As authoritative experts in the Dry Needle technique, we would like to share with you the limitations of the Dry Needle Technique and how due to these limitations Dry Needle actually becomes acupuncture. This leads to what many in the acupuncture profession believe is the unethical practice of acupuncture by those with no training and no understanding of the principles of acupuncture.

Let us be the first to tell you, the muscle twitch is not always elicited. In my experience the trapezius muscle is the only one that may have a reliable expectation of getting an elicited "muscle twitch" from the needle intervention. Even so it is not always the case. After the trapezius the muscle twitch may be a rare, infrequent, or unpredictable event. The sole purpose of the "dry needle technique" is to elicit this muscle twitch response.

So what happens when the practitioner has difficulty eliciting a muscle twitch response, which is a rare, infrequent, or unpredictable? They begin to use more aggressive and painful needle intervention (which is concerning to the acupuncture profession due to the pain suffered and potential turn off of patients who are unable to distinguish between acupuncture and dry needle). The dry needle practitioner uses more needles, they retain the needles, they use distal point needling, and they use traditional acupuncture points.

Due to the limitations of the Dry Needle Technique the dry needle practitioner has in essence stopped doing dry needle and in reality has begun practicing acupuncture. We see this over and over every day in every picture posted by the dry needle practitioners. With retained needles, or distal needles far away from the location of pain, or hundreds of needles tracking along the course of a muscle, we see the departure from dry needle into the practice of acupuncture, albeit in its most ignorant and unlearned form.

This is where the dry needle technique becomes the unethical practice of acupuncture. This is the difference between 25 hours of training in a weekend class versus the minimal 2,000 plus hours in a properly accredited, properly supervised didactic and clinical environment necessary for the licensed acupuncturist.

This is the concern of the acupuncture profession. The Dry Needle technique is the pandora's box and open door that allows a practitioner to perform acupuncture in ignorance of the principles of acupuncture. Not only is the practitioner ignorant but so too is the patient.

As licensed professionals in the acupuncture profession we can assure our patients of our knowledge of the science behind our medicine. We examine, observe, diagnose, and intervene according to the classification of this science and medicine. The knowledge and practice of this science is what makes acupuncture as effective and popular as it is. It takes time, patience, study, and experience to learn.

This letter is to offer our authoritative experience on the dry needle technique to our fellow medical professionals. It is with encouragement that we recommend those who wish to practice acupuncture to learn the complete program in a properly accredited and supervised acupuncture institution.

"To the novice, acupuncture seems simple. The experienced know otherwise."

Acupuncture Physiology, Dry Needling, and Cold

Acupuncture physiology; studied, observed, and intervened upon over the course of millennia is one of the most extraordinary and consistent explanations of the human condition. This marvelous engineering construct of human physiology, health, and disease is made up of several components, such as the study and classification of the internal organs and their five element relationships of harmony (health and balance) and disharmony (disease, pain, illness), yin / yang, and Qi.

A major component of acupuncture physiology that is unique and reigns supreme above all other medical health constructs is the study of cold. "Shan Han Lun" compiled by Zhang Zhongjing sometime before the year 220 AD is the seminal work and study of cold induced disease. In this work, cold and the invasion of cold into the body is studied and observed as it passes (or is expelled) from the superficial channels and structures of the body into the deeper channels and organs. Corresponding signs and symptoms will manifests at each of these levels. The skilled acupuncture and oriental medicine practitioner will be able to identify these levels of cold through observation of the pulse, tongue, palpitation, and other means during the examination of the patient.

Cold is a major factor in muscle pathology of dry needling. In the previous article "Acupuncture's Dry Needle Technique /Muscle Trigger Point" eight mechanisms were explained in the pathology of muscle trigger points. The first mechanism of a trigger point is that muscle becomes shortened. The fourth mechanism of trigger points in muscles is inhibited circulation of blood and oxygen through muscle tissue.

Exposure to cold or the use of cold upon a muscle with knots can be the triggering event of pain, or the stabilizing event of pain (meaning it will keep one in a painful condition, for a longer period of time). In a muscle that is shortened with knots, cold will constrict and shorten the muscle even further. Cold also constricts blood vessels which further inhibits the circulation of blood through tissue already deficient from the presence of knots. This mechanism is confirmed by the use of ice in the case of sprains or strains. Ice is applied to restrict blood vessels and the circulation of blood, stemming the hemorrhage and keeping the swelling down.[xvi]

Acupuncture physiology is the foremost medical system that explains in detail the effect of cold in the body. As part of Acupuncture's Dry Needle Technique /Muscle Trigger Point Therapy the skilled practitioner of acupuncture and oriental medicine will be able to advise their patient whether they are susceptible to cold induced disease, identify the exposure event of cold that caused their pain, and steps to avoid exposure to cold. As part of their dry needling technique the acupuncturist may use warming therapy, included but not limited to the use of moxibustion, herbs, and warm food recommendations.

[xvi] http://www.healthline.com/health/chronic-pain/treating-pain-with-heat-and-cold#Cold3

The Needle as a Therapeutic and Diagnostic Tool

The purpose of Acupuncture's Dry Needle technique is of course to obtain a therapeutic effect and benefit. There can also be information provided of the patient's condition from the performance of acupuncture's dry needle technique.

Scope of practice advisory - Much of the following discussion is limited to the expertise and scope of acupuncture and oriental medicine. Those practicing outside of this scope are not qualified to offer diagnosis or examination upon patients without proper education and licensing requirements to practice acupuncture.

Mentioned before about the limitations of the dry needle technique is the frequent inability to elicit a muscle twitch from the needle. One particular reason observed from practice by the author may be dryness or dehydration of the muscle due to the presence of heat. This is particularly noticeable when needling the trapezius.

During the push and pull of acupuncture's dry needle technique upon the trapezius the practitioner will get a sense of dehydration and dryness of the muscle. Akin to a pulse diagnosis, the needle insertion will have a choppy, irregular feel to it. There will be combination of resistance and vacuity as the needle passes through levels and strands of dry stringy muscle fiber. Perhaps the trigger point, neuro-muscular junction is more unresponsive due to mineral and fluid deficiency, but it may take more effort to elicit a twitch response.

Dryness or dehydration in a muscle due to heat will further be confirmed through the comprehensive examination performed by the acupuncturist. Their given diagnosis may be something along the lines of blood and body deficiency to heat, which will be evident in pulse and tongue as well as visual inspection of the patient. There may be excessive reddening or heat macules upon the chest, neck, and back from overexposure to sun or internal rising of heat.

Other correspondent signs of dehydration may be the affliction of muscle cramps throughout the body suffered by the patient. This is a wind condition, another indication of blood and body fluid deficiency. Or the patient frequently has a dry mouth and tongue. The acupuncturist may offer herbs or other remedies to supplement blood and body fluids.

The Quadratus Lumborum is a muscle that will have a dense "sticky" feeling if it is very tightly constricted and unbalanced. The more dense or sticky it feels to the practitioner, the more likely the patient may feel they are receiving an "injection" of some sorts from the acupuncture needle. Even though this is a quick needle technique without retention of the needle, the patient may feel as if the needle is still retained after its removal. It is important to assure the patient the needle has been removed as they may be tentative in movement for whatever the next procedure the practitioner has ready for them.

Death by Diagnosis
Stenosis, Bulging Discs, Lower Back Pain, Oh My!

"Death by Diagnosis" - a psychological effect whereby a patient's condition worsens after being given a negative diagnosis or prognosis from MRI imaging, X-ray, or doctor.

Many patients who come to acupuncture seek relief for lower back pain, which is not surprising as lower back pain accounts for the second leading cause of office visits to physicians[xvi] in general. Upon entering the health care system many patients will undergo MRI or Xray imaging examinations to help confirm or make the diagnosis in regards to their condition. While these examinations are useful diagnostic tools they can sometimes cause needless discouragement in regards to the prognosis of the patient's condition.

The reason is that many normal, healthy people have abnormalities like disc, stenosis, or other conditions in their lumbar spine, while exhibiting no symptomatic effects of from such conditions. In spite of the abnormality there is no pain and no limitation in function. "MR images in adults younger than 60 years with no history of back pain or sciatic, Boden and colleagues found that approximately half had bulging discs and degenerative discs and nearly a quarter had herniated discs. In adults older than 60 years, all findings were even more common, and both bulging and degenerative discs were almost ubiquitous. Similar studies by others have produced remarkably similar results."[xvi][xvi]

Abnormalities of the spine are often normal processes of life and aging and may not be the cause of the back pain at all. Myofascial (muscle related) issues may be at the forefront of any lower back in spite of structural abnormalities lingering beneath. Quite often patients who have received discouraging reports vis a vis their imaging examinations or doctors can get relief from acupuncture.

Acupuncturist perform a multitude of interventions for pain including stretching exercises, cupping, moxibustion, and a wide variety of acupuncture techniques including dry needle. Often dry needling is combined seamlessly with traditional acupuncture procedures and techniques. Due to the use of dry needle upon sensitive trigger point areas and the repeated push and pull required by the technique, dry needle may be more painful than traditional acupuncture. In the hands of a qualified skilled acupuncturist dry needle can be optimally performed with minimal discomfort.

When favorable results are achieved through acupuncture it is a cause for celebration. It shows what is possible and achievable in spite of the structural abnormalities. If you have full function and no pain it is a cause for optimism. Do not let your diagnosis get you discouraged.

[xvi] Cypress BK. Characteristics of physician visits for back symptoms: a national perspective. Am J Public Health. 1983;73:389–395. doi: 10.2105/AJPH.73.4.389

[xvi] Jensen, M. C., et. al., "Magnetic Resonance Imaging of the Lumbar Spine in People Without Back Pain." N Eng J Med 1994, 331 (200), 69-73. Jarvik, J. J., et. al., "Longitudinal Assessment of Imaging and Disability of the Back (LAIDBack) Study: Baseline Data." Spine 2001, 26 (10), 1158-1166.

[xvi] Travis, Russell "Abnormal Findings in Normal People" http://www.aadep.org/ article Dec 2009

Acupuncture Muscle Trigger Point and Oriental Medicine Sports Therapy Lebron James and Game One of the 2014 NBA Finals. A case study on dehydration, cold, and the use of ice.

It is of course difficult to ascertain the internal condition of professional basketball player Lebron James during game one of the 2014 NBA finals, in which he developed debilitating muscle cramps that led to his premature removal from the game. There was however one piece of evidence that may have contributed to his condition. It was the use of ice upon his body during intermissions in play of the game.

It was game one of the 2014 NBA finals in San Antonio, Texas. Lebron James was the star player for the visiting Miami Heat. An unforeseen technical glitch occurred in the arena though. The air conditioning stopped functioning and it became hot. Temperatures reached as high as 90 degrees during the game. [i]

Due to the vigorous nature of the game, players were no doubt sweating profusely and losing body fluid. Lebron James received intravenous fluids during the game and trainers placed ice on his neck to cool his core body temperature. In pictures ice is seen placed on his left leg.[ii] The working diagnosis as to the cause of Lebron James cramps was "dehydration". [iii] Certainly dehydration should be considered a factor in getting cramps. However, an alternate explanation thus far unmentioned was the use of ice.

In the preeminent procedures and principles of Acupuncture and Oriental Medicine, cold is factor that can trigger pain or stabilize a painful condition (meaning that it can keep one in a painful condition for longer period of time). "Cold contracts and obstructs and this often causes pain."[iv] In the mechanism of muscle trigger points, where muscles are shortened due to the presence of knots, the use of ice will contract the muscle and shorten it even more.

Acupuncture Muscle Trigger Point therapy [v]

Trigger points are knots or nodules located in muscle tissue. The first mechanism that occurs due to the presence of knots in the muscle tissue is that the muscle becomes "SHORTENED". The analogy is if you take a piece of rope and tie it into a knot, it will shorten the length of that rope. Knots (Trigger Points) are clusters of fascia which tangle up and shorten the length of muscle.

The second mechanism that occurs due to trigger points is that they add increased tension and strain on the tendons. If the muscle is shortened it adds more strain on the tendon. A stretched and tightened tendon will likely rub with increased friction against adjacent tissues. Tendinitis (inflammation of the tendon) and muscle strains/ sprains are the most common injuries and diagnosis resulting from shortened muscles.

The third mechanism that occurs due to the presence of trigger points is the range of motion of the joint or limb will be decreased. The pull and strain from the shortened muscle and tightened tendon, simply will not allow the full range of motion of the joint or limb. When we do accidentally twist our foot or limb beyond its inhibited range of motion, a muscle sprain or strain will occur. Further damage such as a tear can also occur.

Fourth mechanism that occurs due to the presence of trigger points is that they inhibit the circulation of blood and oxygen to the muscle tissue. Blood and oxygen have a harder time circulating through the cluster of knotted tissue and fascia. The muscle becomes dehydrated. Dr. Hyungsuk Choi of Samra Acupuncture Center states the muscle tissue becomes a "Beef Jerky" like consistency, very dry and stringy. [vi]

Fifth Mechanism, a muscle that is dry and stringy with trigger points is unable to be strengthened. To strengthen, you must restore it to its normal length, tenderness, and pliability first.

Sixth Mechanism, the trigger point is painful upon palpation. The pain felt does not have to be local to the trigger point area. Pain will refer to points where the muscle attaches and inserts. Many painful diseases are actually located distantly away from where the trigger point occurs.

Seventh Mechanism is that trigger points can be present without any pain or physical complaint. Until a triggering event occurs (like accident, injury, or exposure to cold and ice). There may be no physical complaint even though the trigger point is present.

Eighth Mechanism: Peripheral Nerve Impingement. A shortened muscle/ stretched tendon may pinch on the nerves at the periphery (outside of the spinal column) causing radiating pain, numbness, or tingling down arms or joints. This is a more favorable prognosis as muscle stretching / tendon relaxation will eliminate the nerve impingement.

The use of ice and dehydration.

The most commonly used form of ice as therapy occurs after a muscle strain / sprain like a twisted ankle. When a joint or limb accidently move beyond its normal range of motion, micro blood vessels in the tissues tear and hemorrhaging of blood and body fluid begin to cause swelling. The use of ice is applied to restrict blood vessels and the circulation of blood, stemming the hemorrhage and keeping the swelling down.[vii] This same mechanism of using ice can exasperate a dehydrated condition, further depleting blood, body fluid, and oxygen to tissues.

Dehydration

According to the Mayo clinic "overuse of a muscle, dehydration, muscle strain or simply holding a position for a prolonged period of time may result in a muscle cramp. In many cases, however, the exact cause of a muscle cramp isn't known."[viii] Other causes may be due to inadequate blood supply, nerve compression, and mineral depletion.

Dehydration in Oriental Medicine

The initial diagnosis a practitioner of acupuncture and oriental medicine would probably make in the case of dehydration is blood and body fluid deficiency. "The main function of Blood is that of nourishing the body… Besides providing nourishment, Blood also has a moistening function. Blood ensures that body tissues do not dry out."[ix] The liver stores and rejuvenates blood when we rest. When we are active the Liver sends blood to the sinews and tissues. "Deficiency of the liver blood deprives the tendons of nourishment and thus stirs up a deficiency wind type in the interior."[x] A muscle spasm or cramp is classified as a wind condition in oriental medicine. The analogy of blood deficiency generating wind, is when barometric pressure drops, it foretells stormy windy conditions. "When blood fails to nourish the limbs and tendons, there may be numbness of the limbs and spasms of the tendons."[xi]

Cold can also be a cause of dehydration as it blocks the mechanisms of transport to and from the tissues, especially in one who is yang deficient and unable to use the body's resources to warm up. "Pain with a cold sensation and preference for warmth often occurs in the head, lumbar, epigastric, and abdominal regions. It is caused by cold blocking the collaterals or lack of warmth and nourishment in the zang-fu organs and meridians due to deficiency of yang qi."[xii]

The analogy of cold causing dehydration is the Antarctica, an extremely cold and dry environment. Cold dehydration may be identified with symptoms of cold hands and feet when the weather drops or from exposure to air conditioning. Growing up in a cold environment may make one susceptible to cold influences. Cold dehydration can be exasperated from under dressing in cold weather, ice cold drinks, going barefoot on cold ground surfaces, swimming in cold water.

If I were to ask Lebron James one question, it would be whether he easily gets cold hands or feet when the weather turns cold. An athlete of his caliber I would expect the answer to be 'no'. However he grew up and lives in Cleveland, Ohio along the banks of Lake Erie which gets extremely cold and windy in the winter. So maybe he has some deep lingering cold? If so, then the use of ice on him should be contraindicated.

Oriental Medicine Therapies for the treatment of dehydration, muscle cramps, and cold.

Warm Therapy

In the preeminent procedures and principles of acupuncture and oriental medicine, if cold is identified during the examination of the patient, then the use of cold as therapy in the form of herbs or otherwise is contraindicated. Warming herbs or procedures such as (moxibustion) are used to counter the influence of cold.

Oriental Medicine Therapy

In the case of dehydration causing muscle cramps herbal medicine such as the formula Shao Yao Gan Cao Tang can be used. This two herb formula of blood and Qi tonic herbs "softens the liver, moderates painful spasms, and alleviates pain. Indications for the use of this formula are for irritability, slight chills, spasms of the calf muscles, and lack of coating on the tongue. There may also be cramps in the hands and abdominal pain. This formula is used for when the inappropriate use of sweating has injured the liver blood or yin. Today it is used for any type of pain in the calves with blood deficiency or injury to the fluids. The irritability and lack of tongue coating are attributed to injury to the yin. The spasms, cramps, and abdominal pain are typical spasmodic, wind - like manifestations of Liver blood deficiency."[xiii]

Ginseng is another herb that can support the body against dehydration. One of its many uses is for "generating fluids and stopping thirst, in cases when the qi and fluids have been injured by high fever and profuse sweating."[xiv]

Acupuncture Muscle Trigger Point Techniques

For muscle trigger point release I practice the Korean Acupuncture techniques of VST Acupuncture (Vertex Synchronizing Technique) and Korean Kinetic Acupuncture.

Saam Acupuncture

Spleen Jungguk - the energetic aspect of the Spleen Jungguk is to bring warmth and moisture within. The harmonized technique of adding the Small Intestine helps to generate blood.

Lung Jungguk - The energetic aspect of the Lung Jungguk is to add cool and moisture within, making it useful for heat dehydration.

i http://www.foxsports.com/nba/story/air-conditioning-malfunction-game-1-san-antonio-att-center-lebron-james-tim-duncan-060514

ii

iii http://espn.go.com/nba/playoffs/2014/story/_/id/11048753/lebron-james-salty-solution

iv Maciocia, Giovanni, "The Foundations of Chinese Medicine", Churchill Livingstone, 1989, page 183

v Excerpts taken from "Saam Korean Acupuncture: Advanced Combinations" copyright 2013 by Evan Mahoney

vi Choi, Hyungsuk, Hamsoa Childrens Hospital, Los Angeles, Korea. This quote was taught to me verbally by Dr. Choi during my training under him at Samra Acupuncture Center.

vii http://www.healthline.com/health/chronic-pain/treating-pain-with-heat-and-cold#Cold3

viii http://www.mayoclinic.org/diseases-conditions/muscle-cramp/basics/causes/con-20014594

ix Maciocia, Giovanni, "The Foundations of Chinese Medicine", Churchill Livingstone, 1989, page 50

x Xinnong, Cheng editor, "Chinese Acupuncture and Moxibustion", Foreign Languages Press Beijing, 1999 sixth printing 2005, page 277-278 316.

xi Ibid., 316

xii Xinnong, Cheng editor, "Chinese Acupuncture and Moxibustion", Foreign Languages Press Beijing, 1999 sixth printing 2005, page 277-278

xiii Bensky, Dan and Barolet, Randall, "Chinese Herbal Medicine, Formulas and Strategies" Eastland Press, 1990, pgs 252 -253

xiv Bensky, Dan and Gamble, Andrew, "Chinese Herbal Medicine, Materia Medica, revised edition", Eastland Press, 1990, pg 314

VST (Vertex Synchronizing Technique) Acupuncture

VST acupuncture founded by Dr. Jonghwa Lee is a Korean Acupuncture Trigger Point Release Technique. VST acupuncture measures range of motion across the three planes (transverse, sagittal, coronal) of the neck, shoulder, lower back, and hip to identify affected antagonist muscles. VST then utilizes trigger point acupuncture to release the antagonistic muscle to restore range of motion and give pain relief.

VST has applications across the entire body structures but for purposes of this paper VST will be used only for the vertexes of the neck/ shoulder, lower back and hips.

VST Acupuncture Range of Motion Analysis

Neck Range of Motion Analysis

Cervical Forward flexion - Sagittal Plane Analysis - Normal Range of Motion is 50 degrees[i]

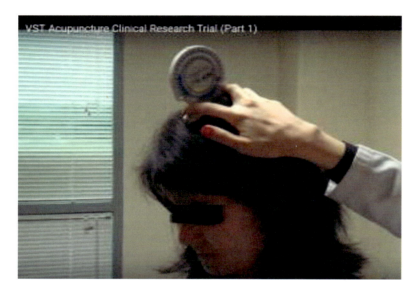

Cervical Neck Extension - Sagittal Plane Analysis - normal range of motion is 60 degrees[ii]

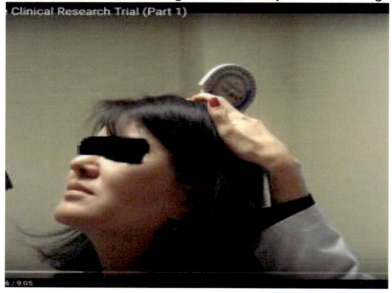

In the cervical neck extension and flexion the primary affected muscles are suboccipitals with corresponding acupoints DU 15, 16 and Urinary Bladder 10, sternocleidomastoid with corresponding acupoints Large Intestine 16,17,18, and upper trapezius with corresponding acupoints GB 21.[iii]

Neck Lateral Bending (left right) - normal range of motion is 45 degrees[iv]

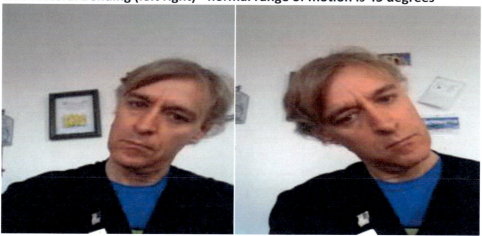

Neck Rotation (left right) - normal range of motion is 80 degrees[v]

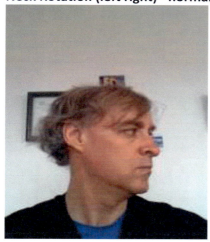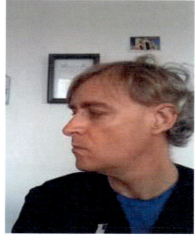

Shoulder Range of Motion

External Rotation - Transverse Plane Analysis - normal range of motion is 90 degrees
Normal motion the arms should reach back to touch the table. If there is restricted range of motion the subscapularis and pectoralis minor muscles are the affected antagonist muscle. There is a special way to needle the subscapularis trigger points but in general acupoints Urinary Bladder 41-43 will be the points chosen. For the Pectoralis Minor, trigger point surrounding LU 2 will be chosen.[vi]

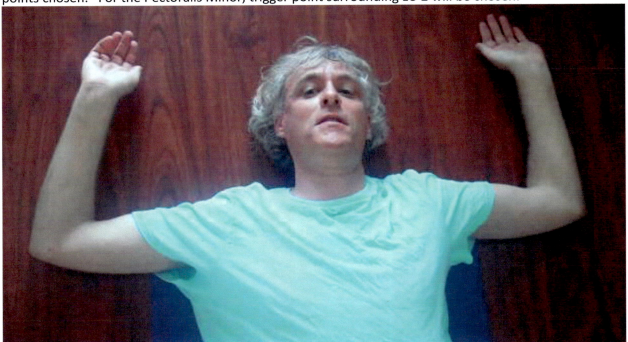

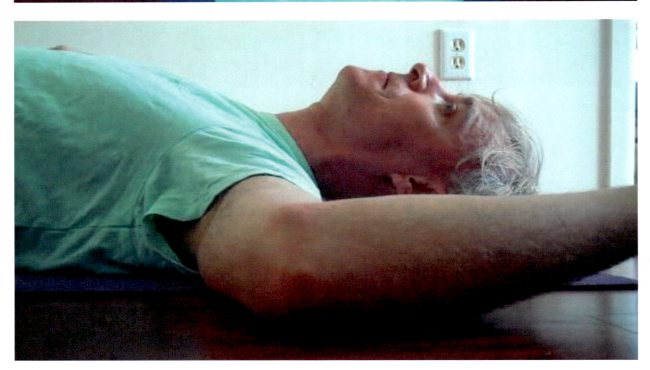

Internal Rotation - Transverse Plane Analysis - normal range of motion is 90 degrees

Normal range of motion the arms should reach forward to touch the table. If there is restricted range of motion the infraspinatus and teres minor are the affected antagonist muscles. Trigger points in the area of acupoints Small Intestine 9 and 11 will be selected.[vii]

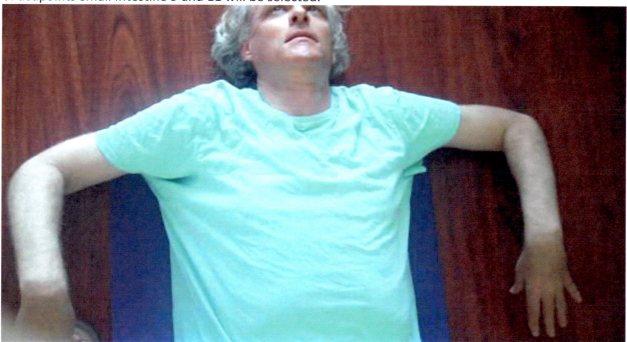

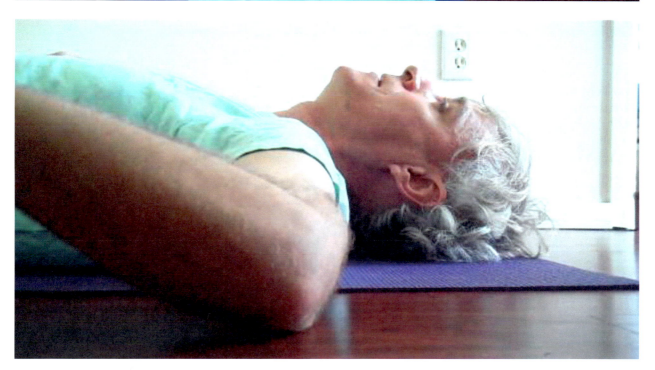

Arm Length - Coronal Plane Analysis

If one arm is shorter than the other the latismuss dorsi and teres major muscles are restricting the full range of motion. Use trigger point acupuncture to this muscles in the area of acupoints Gall Bladder 22 and 23.[viii]

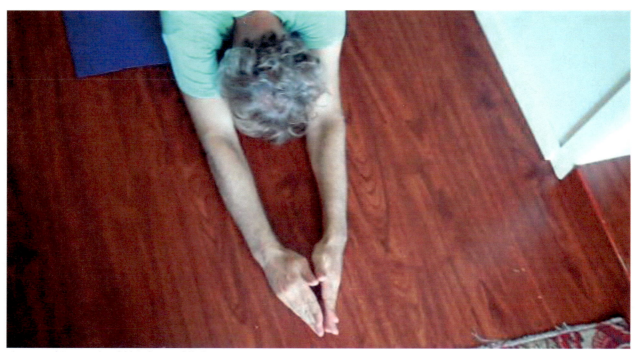

Figure 3 This test should be done while lying on a treatment table.

Shoulder Abduction Apley's Scratch Test

Prime mover Deltoid and Supraspinatus. Affected antagonist muscle latismuss dorsi, pectoralis minor.

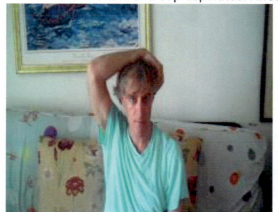
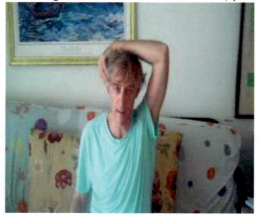

VST Acupuncture Lower Back and Hip Range of Motion Analysis

Hip

Internal Rotation - Transverse Plane Analysis - normal range of motion is 40 degrees

If there is restricted range of motion for internal rotation of the hips the Gluteus Medius, Piriformis, and Tensor Fascia Muscles are the affected antagonist muscles. Use trigger point acupuncture in the area of Gall Bladder 29.[ix]

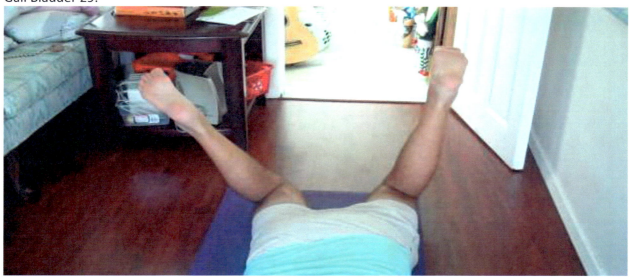

External Rotation - Transverse Plane Analysis - normal rotation is 45 degrees

If there is restricted range of motion of external range of motion Oblique Abdominal, Sartorius, and Psoas are the affected antagonist muscles. Use trigger point acupuncture in the area of Spleen 14, 15 (Oblique Abdominal), Stomach 31 (Sartorius), and GB 26 (Psoas). [x]

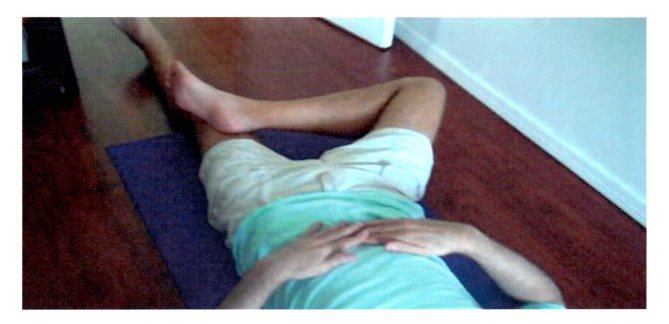

Leg Length Difference - Coronal Plane Analysis

During the leg length difference test the practitioner should also view the level of the hips and pelvic girdle. If one leg is shorter the gluteus maximus muscle is contracted. The level of the buttocks on the shortened side should be higher than the longer leg length side. Using trigger point acupuncture to acupoint area Gall Bladder 30.[xi]

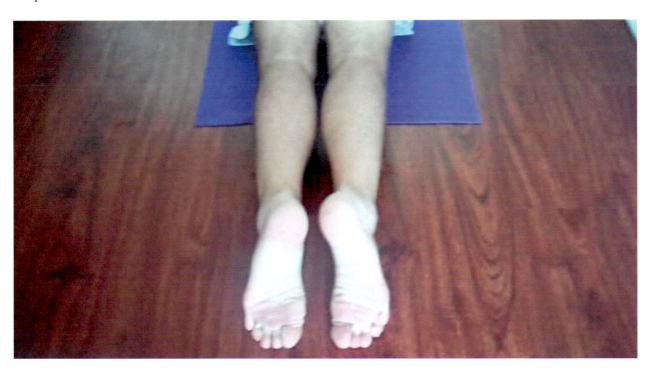

Lateral Bending - Coronal Plane Analysis -normal range of motion is 25 degrees
Affected muscle Quadratus Lumborum

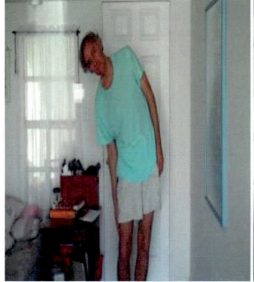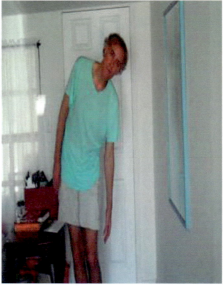

VST Acupuncture for Neck

Order of Needle Insertion

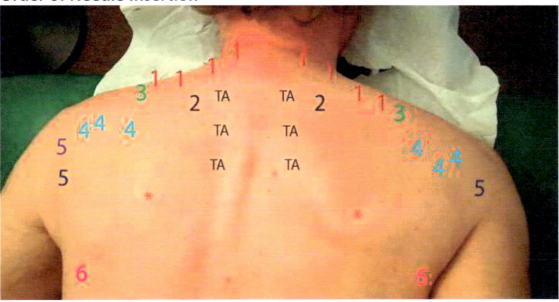

The following needles can be retained.

1. **Trapezius**
2. **Levetar Scapulae**
3. **Supraspinatus**
4. **Infraspinatus**
5. **Teres Minor**

6. **Teres Major -if necessary (if arm length is difference) do not retain needles.**

7. **TA = Traditional Acupuncture** - Traditional Acupuncture points can be woven in with VST. In fact VST is not a dry needle technique because the needles are retained. (Dry Needle only involves quick insertion and withdrawal of the needle). Therefore VST and acupuncture are seamlessly interwoven techniques.

   The acupuncture practitioner has the choice to perform other techniques of their choosing (should they wish) to coincide with VST.

*Subscapularis - if done, should be done 1st with insertion and quick withdrawal, see image below. This is because in order to needle the subscapularis we need to position the patients arm behind them. This will cause the Scapulae to wing out. Needle insertion is 1.5 cun obliquely (pointing the needle in the direction of the scapular wall. X's mark the spot of needle insertion at level T5- T7.

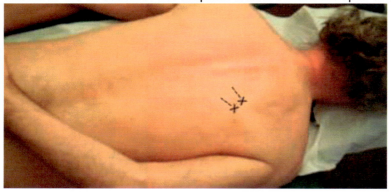

VST Acupuncture for Lower Back

This is a practitioners choice. The practitioner can needle Ashi points across the wide area of the Gluteus Muscles, Iliac Crest, and Hips. VST is further supplemented with traditional acupuncture points of the Urinary Bladder, Gall Bladder, and extra points located in the lower back, gluteal region.

My Capstone Project for completion of my Doctoral Degree

Presented here is a study of VST acupuncture in four sections relating to pain of acute and chronic nature and pain located in the Lower Back and Neck.

Dr. Jonghwa Lee is the creator of VST Acupuncture. He completed his M.S and Ph.D., in Oriental Medicine, at Kyung Hee University, Seoul, Korea. He is the founder of VST institute and Bluehill Clinic with six branches in Seoul, Korea.

It was my honor and privilege to work closely with Dr. Lee in the clinic and classroom didactic education during Samra's doctoral program.

VST Acupuncture Study

Dr. Evan Mahoney, Dr. Heejoo Kim, Dr. Young June Yoon, Dr .Christie Chon, Dr. Jonghwa Lee, Dr. Hyungsuk Choi.   From Samra University/ Emperor's College Doctoral Studies Program June 2011

Background: This is the combined results of the VST Acupuncture pilot study undertaken by the researchers as part of their doctoral program capstone studies at Emperor's College, completed June 2011.   This paper is the combined results of the four pilot studies on VST acupuncture.

Purpose: The purpose of the four pilot studies was to test the efficacy of VST acupuncture on lower back, neck and shoulder pain, in both chronic and acute cases.

Methodology: There were 25 participants in the combined pilot studies who qualified as either acute or chronic, low back and neck and shoulder pain patients. Eight of these patients had both low back, neck and shoulder pain and were included in both a neck or low back study.

1. There were four participants in the **Lower Back Pain/ Acute** pilot study.
2. There were thirteen participants in the **Lower Back Pain/ Chronic** pilot study.
3. There were seven participants in the **Neck and Shoulder Pain/ Acute** pilot study.
4. There were twelve participants in the **Neck and Shoulder Pain/ Chronic** pilot study.

The researchers gathered data on these patients using the VAS (Visual Analog Scale) filled out by the patient and range of motion tests of the lower back, neck, and shoulder. These measurements were conducted before and after the administration of VST acupuncture.

Conclusions:

VAS pain scale:
1. **Lower back pain/ Acute cases** - The average decrease in pain (measured by VAS) after the administration of VST acupuncture was 8.25%. The p-value of the VAS for the group before and after treatment was 0.198.
2. **Lower back pain/Chronic cases** - The average decrease in pain (measured by the VAS) after the administration of VST acupuncture was 57.45 %. The p-value of the VAS for the group before and after treatment was 0.0021.

3. **Neck and Shoulder pain / Acute cases** - The average decrease in pain (measured by the VAS) after the administration of VST acupuncture was 30.2%. The p-value of the VAS for the group before and after treatment was 0.041

4. **Neck and Shoulder pain / Chronic cases** - The average decrease in pain (measured by the VAS) after the administration of VST acupuncture was 48.3%. The p-value of the VAS for the group before and after treatment was 0.001

Range of motion tests:

1. **Lower back pain/ Acute cases** – There were improvements in range of motion of the lower back and external rotation of the hips both sides, leg length difference, and lateral bending to the left side. The external rotation of the right hip measured a statistically relevant p-value of .044.

2. **Lower back pain/ Chronic cases** - There were improvements in range of motion of the lower back and hip joint areas for internal and external rotation of the hips both sides, leg length difference, and lateral bending to the left side.

3. **Neck and Shoulder pain/ Acute cases** - There were small improvements on the averages of internal and external rotation of the shoulder both sides, arm length difference, and lateral bending to the left side. Only internal rotation of the left shoulder had a P-value of significance at 0.377138153. All other T-paired test values came as statistically irrelevant.

4. **Neck and Shoulder pain/ Chronic cases** - Range of motion of the neck and shoulder area improved on cervical flexion, lateral bending to right side, and external rotation of left shoulder in degree ($P \leq 0.001$). Internal rotation of left and right shoulder and external rotation of left and right shoulder improved in degree ($P \leq 0.05$). Length differences of left and right arm decreased ($P \leq 0.001$) and ROM of internal and external rotation differences of left and right shoulder joints are reduced and balanced after VST acupuncture.

Filming of procedure: The researcher has filmed the examination and treatment procedures of the VST acupuncture technique. The video clips can be viewed online at youtube.com under the following links.

http://www.youtube.com/watch?v=1cWJW48WH5s - video 1
http://www.youtube.com/watch?v=wpBMNb_4e_Q - video 2
http://www.youtube.com/watch?v=x3uYu7hRGHA – video 3

Chapter 1

Definitions/ Persons relevant to VST acupuncture

VST (vertex synchronizing technique) was developed by Dr. Jonghwa Lee, who practices in both Korea and the United States. VST is an acupuncture technique used to rebalance and align the body according to its tensegrity. The use of Sagittal, Coronal, and Transverse analysis of range of motion and body position, identifies which muscles should be treated with VST acupuncture. VST is applicable across the whole body. VST acupuncture is a synthesis of oriental medicine with modern western musculoskeletal therapy. VST traces the western medical aspect of its technique from the works of Dr. Janet Travell ,

C.Chan Gunn and their work with muscle trigger points and Thomas W. Myers and the application of the tensegrity model.

Tensegrity Model: "is adopted to explain the alignment of our bodies. A typical tensegrity model is made with wooden sticks and rubber bands. Each one of them connected together to form a perfect state of balance with its shape in place. If a single rubber band's tension is uneven for an instant, the whole structure will not be able to hold its balanced shape anymore. The muscles and bones in our body are similar to this structure. Muscles act like the rubber bands and they pull, while the bones like the stick holds the structure. This is how our bodies keep their structural balance ideally, through homeostatsis. [xii]

Neck and Shoulder Vertex: Includes the muscles of the neck and shoulder which are tested for imbalances using range of motion tests and length measurements. The muscles of the neck and shoulder vertex for the purpose of this study are latismus dorsi, trapezius, infraspinatus, supraspinatus, teres minor, teres major, and levator scapulae.

Lower Back Vertex: Includes muscles of the lower back and hip joint which are tested for imbalances using range of motion tests and length measurements. The muscles of the lower back vertex for the purpose of this study are gluteus maximus, medius and minimus, tensor fascia latae, abdominal oblique, and psoas muscle.

Ashi point: In Traditional Chinese Medicine (TCM) lexicon is a term that refers to any area or point upon palpation that elicits pain, tenderness, or vocal response from the patient. (Xinnong, Cheng 1990) States that ashi points are "also called reflexing points, or unfixed points, or tender spots. Chapter 13 of Miraculous Pivot says tender spots can be used as acupuncture points, and this was the primary method for point selection in early acupuncture and moxibustion treatments. Clinically, they are mostly used for pain syndromes." [xiii] The tender area becomes an acupuncture point, even if it is outside the point meridian structures studied in TCM.

Ashi point acupuncture: Needling with an acupuncture needle into an area or point that has elicited tenderness, pain, or vocal response from patient, when the area was palpated. "Tender spots can be used as acupuncture points" [xiv]

Dr. Janet Travell
Dr. Travell is the author of over 100 research studies and her two-volume book <u>Myofascial Pain and Dysfunction: The Trigger Point Manual</u> co authored by David Simons. She was a personal physician to President John F. Kennedy, for his back pain. She did extensive research in the field of muscle trigger point therapy. She discovered that many types of pain were of a myogenic origin. She demonstrated that procaine injection of MTrPs in patients suffering from the pain of myocardial infarction could stop both noncardiac pain of muscle origin and true cardiac pain of coronary insufficiency. The early studies by Dr. Travell and colleagues provided convincing experimental evidence that active myofascial trigger points can be eliminated, or decreased remarkably, by application of vapocoolant spray to the skin over the painful area. [xv]

She used a focused medical history, a meticulous history of the onset of pain, a detailed identification of the pain pattern, a demonstration of the painfully restricted range of motion, and a finger placed unerringly on the exquisitely tender trigger point. Her application of spray and stretch to that muscle (using Fluori-Methane) always produced immediate and impressive, if not complete, relief of pain and restored full range of motion. [xvi]

Dr. C Chan Gunn

Dr. Gunn coined the phrase "The Shortened Muscle Syndrome", whereby muscle shortening is the structural cause of pain. [xvii] Gunn incorporated the use of an acupuncture needle in his technique "Intramusclar Stimulation (IMS)" which focuses on breaking up muscle trigger points. His technique called "dry needling" is done into trigger points to affect the relaxation and lengthening of muscle tissue which reduces myofascial pain and radiculopathy.   By doing range of motion (ROM) testing he is able to identify which muscle is shortened. An area with restricted ROM is indicative of the presence of muscle trigger points. Afterwards when the trigger point has been effectively anesthesized or broken apart, the muscle tissue should be lengthened, relaxed, and not restricting the ROM anymore.

 Dr. Lee incorporates the same needle technique as Gunn, albeit with a different theoretical basis. Travell, Gunn, and Lee all use palpation of muscle tissue to find trigger points, and all focus their therapies on elimination of muscle trigger points to alleviate pain.

Muscle shortening (The shortened muscle syndrome): (Gunn 2008) Muscle shortening is the key to myofascial pain of neuropathic origin. Stated differently myofascial pain cannot exist in absence of muscle shortening, no shortening no pain. Muscle shortening can be palpated as ropey bands within muscle. The bands are seldom limited to a few individual muscles, but are present in groups of muscles according to the pattern of neuropathy. [xviii]

Muscle Trigger Point: "Focal areas of tenderness and pain are often referred to as "trigger points". When pain is primarily in muscles and is associated with multiple tender trigger points, the condition is referred to as myofascial pain syndrome." [xix]

Dry Needle: Use of a needle not designed for injected substances [xx] for use in muscle trigger point therapy. Acupuncture needles are used for this type of therapy. (Gunn 2008) uses a fine solid needle (30 gauge or less) usually 1 or 2 inches long, in a plunger type needle holder. When it enters normal muscle, the needle meets with little resistance, when it pierces a spasm, there is firm resistance and the needle is "grasped" by the spasm. The fine solid needle therefore allows multiple, closely spaced penetrations to be made without excessive tissue damage. [xxi]

Agonist Muscle: Muscle that initiates the action of movement of limb or body part. [xxii]

Antagonist Muscle: Muscle that counters the action of agonist muscle, and creates movement of limb or body part counter to that of the agonist. [xxiii]

Range of Motion: Measuring the capacity of a limb or body to its fullest movement. Active range of motion is how far the patient can move a limb or body movement under their own power. Passive range of motion is how far the limb or body moves with assistance from another person.

Chapter 2

Back ground on VST acupuncture

What is a Muscle Trigger Point? How does it cause pain?

Irregular posture, prolonged stress, and/or trauma can cause muscle to form into knots of conglomerated fascia, nodules, and thickness, which becomes a trigger point. Trigger points can lie latent in the muscle without exhibiting any signs or symptoms of pain, or they can become activated by an event and become painful. Muscles with trigger points have characteristic features of tenderness and pain that sometimes radiates, usually to the muscle origination or insertion point. While a trigger point may exist in the belly of the muscle the pain complaint of the patient might be some distance away.

In the treatment and identification of trigger points, David Simons who co-authored with Travell concludes "One must learn how to find which muscle or muscles need to be palpated, learn what to palpate for, and either develop the skill to treat the pain or find a therapist with that skill. Any muscle with a painfully restricted range of motion and a tender spot that reproduces the patient's pain when compressed likely has a myofascial trigger point". [xxiv]

Muscle Shortening

A consequence of knotting and tangling of muscle trigger point fascia is that muscles become shortened. Gunn explains "Apart from pain and tenderness that may occur within muscle (possibly from the compression of supersensitive nociceptors), neuropathy increases muscle tone and causes concurrent muscle shortening. Muscle shortening can compress intramuscular nociceptors, mechanically stress tendons, their sheaths and attachments, ligaments, bursae, and joints. Compress disc space, injuring the nerve root and causing radiculopathy, create a self perpetuating circle, lead to fiboris and contractures. Muscle shortening causes a large variety of pain syndromes by its relentless pull on various structures. Myofascial pain cannot exist in absence of muscle shortening - no shortening, no pain". [xxv] [xxvi]

What is VST Acupuncture?

"VST acupuncture is devised and based on scientific bio-mechanical aspects. In VST tensegrity model is applied to examine and analyze the body into coronal, transversal, and sagittal plans. Treatment is focused on restoring three dimensional balances of the shoulder, pelvic girdle and the spinal curve. Evaluations of Range Of Motion in the shoulder and hip joint, which are connecting extremities of the trunk, are performed to find restriction of movement before and after treatment. VST acupuncture directly stimulates and separates layers of muscle and fascia in the adhesion area to promote tension to be released. After treatment , ROM and normal length of the muscles will be reinstated. Blood circulation is also improved at the local site. Application of VST treatment will be effective for not only pain symptoms in knees, shoulders, discs, and spinal problems but will be a key asset to determine the biomechanical systemic cause and will also allow affirmative acupuncture treatment in any variety of musculoskeletal conditions". [xxvii]

"Although VST focuses on the myofascial aspect and biomechanical alignment, it is also in harmony with the traditional theories of meridians. VST also complies very well with the concept of traditional muscular meridians and the eight extra meridians in Oriental Medicine. It is greatly influenced from the three Foot Yang muscular meridians, which reach the core area. Foot Yang Ming muscular meridian (channel running along the anterior body), Foot Tai Yang muscular meridian (channel running along the lateral body) are important in diagnosing and treating coronary and transverse plane problems while the three Foot Yin muscular meridians are important in solving sagittal plane problems.

VST acupuncture is relevantly designed with physical examination and its corresponding treatment. The main purpose is emphasized in balanced normalization of all connective tissue including the fascia and the muscle for maintaining tensegrity of the whole body. Tensegrity structures can be ruined by adhesions in muscle or fascia layers causing resistance in their sliding movement and by the tightness of muscles" [xxviii]

Tensegrity Model

The tensegrity model was first coined by Buckminster Fuller in his explanation of spherical structures and forces maintaining stability of structures. "He explored these ideas through studies of the close-packing of spheres and tensile and compressive stabilization models, noting that tension and compression are not opposites, but rather complements that can be found together; when the two forces are harmonious, continuous pull is balanced by equally discontinuous pushing forces. This synergy between compression and tension is what Fuller calls tensegrity, "a system that stabilizes itself mechanically because of the way in which tensional and compressive forces are distributed and balanced within the structure (Ingber 48-9)". [xxix]

"On an anatomical level, the human body provides a good example of a prestressed tensegrity structure. Bones act as struts resisting the pull of tensile muscles, tendons and ligaments. Moreover, the stability of the shape of the body, or its stiffness, of the body is a function of the tone, or prestress, of its muscles (Ingber Lab). As Ingber puts it, "We are 206 compression-resistant bones that are pulled up against the force of gravity and stabilized through a connection with a continuous series of tensile tendons, muscles, and ligaments" (Ingber Lab)." [xxx]

Example of Tensegrity Model of human structure.

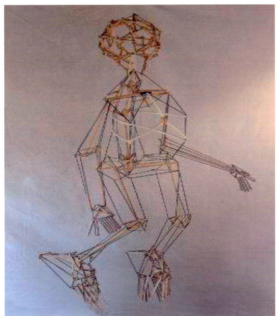

[xxxi]

Tensegrity and Muscle Shortening

Dr. Gunn's "Shortened Muscle Syndrome" nicely applies to the tensegrity model and complications of imbalance. Muscle shortening causes increased stress and pressure upon the tendons and supporting structures that are attached to the shortened muscle. (Dr. Choi) in his explanation of Kinetic acupuncture implies that uneven muscle tension to the sides of the spine causes the spine to pull to the side with the shortened, contracted muscle, which is exerting higher tension. When we treat a patient's back pain, we do not work directly on the spine, but rather on the muscles attached to it. By using acupuncture, we can balance the tension of muscles and eventually obtain the proper stance of the spine. [xxxii]

Like a chain reaction of events, an imbalance in one area can spread to other areas over the whole body. A patient with a history of ankle or foot injury, could develop neck or TMJ problems as balance has shifted and the forces of tensegrity have rebalanced from the ankle, to the knees, hips, back, to the neck and shoulders. In such a case where tensegrity has shifted we will see evidence of imbalance, through difference in extremity length in the coronal plane analysis, pelvic and shoulder joint external and internal rotation differences in the transverse plane analysis, and curvature of the vertebra of the sagittal plane analysis. [xxxiii]

Agonist/ Antagonist Muscles in VST

Every movement in the body has an agonist muscle (muscle initiating the action of movement) and an antagonist (muscle countering the action of movement). We seek to identify and treat the antagonist muscle, which is the muscle that is shortened and is restricting the full range of motion of the limb or body part being moved

Identification of Agonist/ Antagonist Muscles for Low Back Pain in VST

For lower back pain patients we identify differences in tensegrity and the affected agonist muscle through using the coronal plane analysis of measuring leg length differences, and the transverse plane analysis of internal rotation of the hips. Through this analysis we will be able to target the affected muscle tissues. If there is a difference in leg length at the coronal plane we thus identify it as the Glutueas Maximus muscle on the shortened side is contracted and is pulling the pelvis downward [xxxiv] (barring any structural differences in limb length). In this case the Glutueas maximus muscle is the antagonist preventing the hip from its normal range of motion.

In the coronal plane if we find restriction in lateral bending of the trunk then the identified antagonist muscle is the Quadratus Lumburam to the affected side. For hip joint testing in the transverse plane, internal rotation restriction of the hips is correlated to the antagonist muscles Tensor Fascia Latae (TFL) and Glutues Medius muscles of the affected side. For external rotation restriction the antagonists muscle are oblique abdominals, sartorious, and psoas. [xxxv]

Per the analysis from coronal and transverse analysis we will have identified the affected antagonist muscles, that are limiting the ROM. It is these muscles that are contracted and shortened and likely to have trigger points. We treat thus by using acupuncture to release the muscle trigger point.

Identification of Agonist/ Antagonist Muscles for Neck and Shoulder Pain in VST

For neck and shoulder pain patients we identify differences in tensegrity and the affected agonist muscle through using the coronal plane analysis of measuring arm length differences, and the transverse plane analysis of internal rotation of the shoulders. Through this analysis we will be able to target the affected muscle tissues. If there is a difference in arm length at the coronal plane we thus identify it as the Latismus Dorsi muscle on the shortened side is contracted and is pulling the arm downward. In this case the Latismus Dorsi muscle is the antagonist muscle.

For shoulder joint testing in the transverse plane, internal rotation restriction of the shoulder is correlated to the antagonist muscles Infraspinatus and Teres Minor of the affected side. For external rotation restriction of the shoulder the antagonists muscle is subscapularis. Limitations of range of motion to the lateral rotation and bending of the head indicate restriction of the trapezius and levator scapulae muscles with possible involvement of the sternocleidomastoid and scalene muscles.

Per the analysis from coronal and transverse analysis we will have identified the affected antagonist muscles, that are limiting the ROM. It is these muscles that are contracted and shortened and likely to have trigger points. We treat thus by using acupuncture to release the muscle trigger point.

Chapter 3

Results of the Collected Data

The researchers have gathered the following data which follows the VST examination and treatment protocol. The first measure was to get a VAS score taken by the patient before the treatment and then another one after the treatment. Range of motion measurements were taken for the vertexes of the head/neck/ shoulder and lower back/ hip joint areas. The vertex measurements are as follows.

- Head/Neck – forward flexion, extension, lateral bending using an inclinometer taken in degrees.
- Shoulder – internal and external range of motion with inclinometer taken in degrees
- Arm length difference measured in centimeters.
- Lower back – forward flexion, extension, lateral bending using an inclinometer taken in degrees.
- Hips – internal range of motion with inclinometer taken in degrees. External range of motion measured in centimeters between the knee and the table.
- Leg length difference measured in centimeters.

These measurements were taken before and after the treatment. The data presented is a self comparison between the before and after treatments. The following statistics were used in the assessment of this data. T-paired test, averages of Range of Motion and Visual Analog Scale scores, and differences between the before and after treatment measurements.

Evaluation of Statistics
The statistics gathered for this VST acupuncture pilot study were run on Microsoft Excel Spreadsheet. The t-paired tests, means, and standard deviation measurements were all run from the toolbar function application. These statistics were confirmed by a third party evaluator using SPSS software.

I.   **Results from Lower Back Pain / Acute Study**

Description of Patient Subjects

There were four patients who participated in this VST acupuncture pilot study who were qualified as acute back pain patients. Three were female and one male. The patients were all of Korean American ethnicity and were between 29 -59 years old. The patients were recruited through the Korean Daily newspaper in the city of Irvine, California.

Table A. *Demographics of Acute Lower Back Pain patients for VST pilot study*

	Male (n=1)		Female (n=3)		Total (n=4)	
Measure	Mean	S.D	Mean	S.D	Mean	S.D
Age	59	X	40	17	45	17
Korean American Ethnicity	100 %		100 %		100 %	

Table B. *Mean and Standard Deviation differences in VAS Scale, Before and After VST Acupuncture*

Measure		VAS Before Treatment		VAS After Treatment		VAS Mean	P Value
	N	Mean	S.D.	Mean	S.D.	Difference	
Back Pain VAS	4	68.3	[23.6]	60	[25.1]	8.3	0.198

** Significance <0.01, Paired t-test.

Table C. *VAS measure of each patient, before and after treatment and differences between*

Patient number	VAS pain before treatment	VAS pain After treatment	Difference in VAS before and after treatment
1	43	41	2
2	93	97	-4
3	54	52	2
4	83	50	33

The VAS readings were asked before and after the administration of VST acupuncture. The patient was asked to put a check mark on the VAS scale (measuring 100 mm).   The VAS was asked on two separate sheets of paper so the patient was not able to see their before treatment check mark when asked to check their pain on the after the treatment VAS.   The VAS scores are measured in millimeters.

Table D. *Mean Differences in Range of Motion measurements, Before and After VST Acupuncture*

Measure	N	ROM Before Treatment Mean	S.D	ROM After Treatment Mean	S.D	Mean Difference	P- Value
Lumbar Flexion	4	89	[30.7]	80.3	[36.3]	8.7	0.233
Lumbar Extension	4	26.8	[6.24]	24.3	[17.1]	2.5	0.341
Lateral Bending Right Side	4	32.3	[11.4]	32.3	[15.3]	0	0.5
Lateral Bending Left Side	4	27	[4.32]	29	[6.16]	-2	0.309
Difference in Leg Length	4	0.2	[0.18]	0.08	[0.1]	0.13	0.097
Internal Rotation Hips Right Side	4	43.8	[14.4]	47.8 [18.8]		-4	0.180
Internal Rotation Hips Left Side	4	47.5	[14.7]	48.5 [14.1]		-1	0.257
External Rotation Hips Right Side	4	20.6	[4.31]	19 [4.66]		1.68	0.133
External Rotation Hips Left Side	4	22.3	[3.39]	20.6 [4.31]		1.63	0.044

** Significance <0.01, Paired t-test

Table E *Lumbar Flexion measurements of each patient before and after treatment including differences*

Patient number	Lumbar Flexion before treatment	Lumbar Flexion after treatment	Difference of Lumbar flexion
1	130	117	- 13
2	63	76	13
3	68	32	-36
4	95	96	1

Table F *Lumbar Extension measurements of each patient before and after treatment including differences*

Patient number	Lumbar Extension before treatment	Lumbar Extension after treatment	Difference of Lumbar Extension
1	35	48	13
2	20	10	-10
3	25	14	-11

4	27	25	-2

Most of the Range of motion measurements were taken in degrees using an inclinometer, the higher the degree of measurement indicates a higher range of motion and greater degree of flexibility, except for the following. External rotation of hips was measured in centimeters from the difference between the knee and the table. The smaller the number indicates a greater flexibility of external rotation of the hips. The leg length measurements were also taken in centimeters. A measurement of zero means the leg lengths were equal. Numbers other than zero indicate a difference in leg length.

In summary the data gathered on acute low back pain is to measure for differences in the patients ROM of limb and trunk movement, leg length, and patients pain level via the Visual Analog scale. These measurements were taken before the treatment of VST acupuncture was applied and after the treatment.

II.   Results from Low Back Pain / Chronic Study

Description of Patient Subjects

There were thirteen patients who participated in this VST acupuncture pilot study who were qualified as chronic back pain patients. Ten were female and three male. The patients were all of Korean American ethnicity and were between 31-79 years old. The patients were recruited through the Korean Daily newspaper in the city of Irvine, California.

Table G. *Demographics of Chronic Lower Back Pain patients for VST pilot study*

	Male (n=3)	Female (n=10)	Total (n=13)
Measure	Mean	Mean	Mean
Age	58	54	55
Korean American E	100 %	100 %	100 %

Table H. VAS measurement before and after

Measure		VAS Before Treatment		VAS After Treatment		VAS Mean Difference	P Value
	N	Mean	S.D.	Mean	S.D.		
Back Pain VAS	13	49.07	[20.17]	24.00	[24.05]	25.07	0.0021

** Significance <0.01, Paired t-test.

The VAS readings were asked before and after the administration of VST acupuncture. There was significant improvement (58%) after VST treatment. The patient was asked to put a check mark on the VAS scale (measuring 100 mm). The VAS was asked on two separate sheets of paper so the patient was not able to see their before treatment check mark when asked to check their pain on the after the treatment VAS. The VAS scores are measured in millimeters.

Table H. *Mean Differences in Range of Motion measurements, Before and After VST Acupuncture*

Measure	N	ROM Before Mean S.D		ROM After Mean S.D	Mean Difference S.D	P- Value
Lumbar Flexion	13	91.00 [21.65]		95.80 [22.03]	4.80 (10.95)	0.0683
Lumbar Extension	13	27.00 [8.96]		27.70 [9.40]	0.70 (4.58)	0.2982
Lateral Bending (R)	13	27.20 [16.46]		28.20 [14.66]	1.00 (6.05)	0.2813
Lateral Bending (L)	13	29.7 [10.82]		32.4 [9.55]	2.7 (10.34)	0.1767
Difference in Leg Length	13	0.28	[0.32]	0.18 [0.36]	0.10 (0.45)	0.2043
Internal Hip Rotation (R)	13	43.77 [7.17]		45.38 [8.30]	1.61 (6.20)	0.1829
Internal Hip Rotation (L)	13	48.76 [11.12]		47.53 [12.65]	-1.2 (8.35)	0.3025
External Hip Rotation (R)	13	18.21	[6.27]	16.96 [6.08]	-1.25 (2.22)	0.0321
External Hip Rotation (L)	13	17.65 [5.94]		16.07 [6.00]	-1.58 (2.15)	0.0105

** Significance <0.01, Paired t-test

Most of the Range of motion measurements were taken in degrees using an inclinometer, the higher the degree of measurement indicates a higher range of motion, a greater degree of flexibility, except for the following. External rotation of hips was measured in centimeters from the difference between the knee and the table. The smaller the number indicates a greater flexibility of external rotation of the hips. The leg length measurements were also taken in centimeters. A measurement of zero means the leg lengths were equal. Numbers other than zero indicate a difference in leg length.

In summary the data gathered on chronic low back pain is to measure for differences in the patients ROM of limb and trunk movement, leg length, and patients pain level via the Visual Analog scale. These measurements were taken before the treatment of VST acupuncture was applied and after the treatment. As the table shows, most of the ROM has been increased after the VST treatment.

III. Results from Neck and Shoulder Pain / Acute Study

Description of Patient Subjects

There were seven patients who participated in this VST acupuncture pilot study who were qualified as acute neck pain patients. Six were female and one male. The patients were all of Korean American ethnicity and were between 29-68 years old. The patients were recruited through the Korean daily newspaper in the city of Irvine, California.

Table I. *Mean and Standard Deviation differences in VAS Scale, before and after VST Acupuncture*

Measure	N	VAS Before Treatment		VAS After Treatment		VAS Mean	P Value
		Mean	S.D.	Mean	S.D.	Difference	
Neck Pain VAS	7	60.9	[21.3]	30.7	[24.1]	30.2	0,041

***Significance <0.01, paired t-test.

 VAS readings were asked before and after the administration of VST acupuncture. The patients were asked to put a check mark on the VAS scale (measuring 100mm). The VAS was asked on two separate sheets of paper so the patient was not able to see their before treatment check mark when asked to check their pain on the after the treatment VAS. The VAS scores are measured in millimeters.

Table J. *Mean Differences in Range of Motion measurements, Before and After VST Acupuncture*

Measure	N	ROM Before Treatment		ROM After Treatment		Mean Difference	P-Value
		Mean	S.D.	Mean	S.D.		
Neck Flexion	7	52	[15]	61.6	[12.7]	-9.6	0.041
Neck Extension	7	67.4	[11.4]	78.1	[11.6]	-10.7	0.012
Lateral Bending Right	7	47.9	[14.6]	49.1	[13.8]	-1.2	0.344
Lateral Bending Left	7	41.6	[9.78]	49	[13]	-7.4	0.025

Measure	N	ROM Before Treatment		ROM After Treatment		Mean Difference	P-Value
		Mean	S.D.	Mean	S.D.		

Measure	N	ROM Before Treatment		ROM After Treatment		Mean Difference	P-Value
		Mean	S.D.	Mean	S.D.		
External Rotation Right Shoulder	7	79.1	[4.49]	85.7	[8.86]	-6.6	0.045
External Rotation Left Shoulder	7	77.9	[11.7]	84.4	[4.35]	-6.5	0.073

Measure	N	ROM Before Treatment		ROM After Treatment		Mean Difference	P-Value
		Mean	S.D.	Mean	S.D.		
Difference in Arm Length	7	.43	[.49]	.39	[.53]	.04	0.429

***Significance <0.01, paired t-test

The Range of motion measurements were taken in degrees using an inclinometer, the higher the degree of measurement indicates a higher range of motion, a greater degree of flexibility. The difference in arm length was measured in centimeters.

In summery the data gathered on neck pain is to measure for differences in the patient's ROM of limb and trunk movement, arm length, and patents pain via the visual Analog scale. These measurements were taken before the treatment VST acupuncture was applied and after the treatment.

IV.   Results from Neck and Shoulder Pain / Chronic Study

The researcher has had positive results using VST acupuncture for chronic neck and shoulder pain patients.   The average decrease in pain by VAS after the VST acupuncture was 48.3% and the P-value before and after VST acupuncture treatment was 0.001.

ROM of the neck and shoulder area is improved on cervical flexion, lateral bending to right side, and external rotation of left shoulder in degree ($P \leq 0.001$). ROM of the neck and shoulder area improved on internal rotation of left and right shoulder and external rotation of left and right shoulder in degree ($P \leq 0.05$).

Length differences of left and right arm is decreased ($P \leq 0.001$) and ROM of internal and external rotation differences of left and right shoulder joints are reduced and balanced after VST acupuncture.

Chapter 4

Conclusions

I.   Conclusions from Lower Back Pain / Acute study

How effective is the VST acupuncture technique for reducing patient's acute lower back pain and affecting range of motion?

The implications gathered from the data collected in this study of VST acupuncture are that patients suffering from acute low back pain may get pain relief and functional improvement in range of motion of the lower back and hip joint areas. Of the four participants in this study in regards to VAS measurements one had a decrease of pain by 33% while two others had a 2% decrease and one had an increase in pain of 4%.   The average decrease in pain after the administration of VST acupuncture was 8.25 %. The p-value for the group in regards to VAS before and after treatment was 0.198 which is statistically irrelevant.

For range of motion of the lower back and hip joint areas there were improvements in the averages of internal and external rotation of the hips both sides, leg length difference, and lateral bending to the left side.   The external rotation of the left hip measured a statistically relevant p-value figure of 0.044. There was no change in the average of lateral bending to the right side, and a decrease in Range of motion on forward flexion and extension of the hips.

It is difficult to draw conclusions from the data gathered on why patients responded the way they did to the VST acupuncture treatment.   This is partly due to the low number of participants in this clinical pilot study. When looking at range of motion measurements compared to VAS measurements there is some puzzling contradictions.

- Patient number 4 registered a 33% improvement in pain between before and after treatments. While there was a great jump in improvement of pain their range of motion on lumbar flexion and extension were virtually unchanged as were their other range of motion measurements.
- Patient number 2 had a 13 degree improvement in lumbar flexion, a 10 degree lessening of lumbar extension and had a pain increase of 4%.
- Patient number 3 had a decrease in lumbar flexion of 36 degrees and a decrease of lumbar extension of 11 degrees and still improved 2% in their pain.

These contradictions will need to be looked at in any future studies of VST acupuncture.
One advantage of conducting a study on VST acupuncture over other types of acupuncture for research is that the VST can incorporate a more individualistic patient treatment and still conform to the standards of clinical study. Every patient is measured with the same range of motion tests, but VST treats the muscles that are imbalanced. For a general study on lower back pain using the range of motion procedures and measurements outlined above, the researcher can treat according to muscle imbalances that differ between patients and still remain in a homogenous clinical type of setting.

II.   Conclusions from Lower Back Pain / Chronic study

How effective is the VST acupuncture technique for reducing patient's chronic lower back pain and affecting range of motion?
In the sample of participants VST acupuncture was able to improve average patient's pain level by 58% according to the VAS measurements. The T-pared test score for before and after the treatment was 0.0021, making the data gathered statistically relevant.

For the range of motion measurements there were improvements on the averages of internal and external rotation of the hips both sides, leg length difference, and lateral bending to the left side. Even though data show the some improvements of the ROM and significant improvement of VAS, the results of this VST pilot study must be determined also as inconclusive. The sample size was not of a sufficient size. With only thirteen participants in the study the data gathered is not statistically relevant. The implications gathered from the data that was collected are that VST may offer pain relief to patients suffering from chronic low back pain.

It must be noted that this VST study on chronic lower back pain was part of a broader and simultaneous study on VST for acute back pain, acute and chronic neck pain. These other studies operated under the exact same procedure and may draw more conclusive or affirmative results than this study on chronic lower back pain.

III.   Conclusions from Neck and Shoulder Pain / Acute study

In the sample of participants VST acupuncture was able to improve patient's pain level by 30.1% according to the VAS measurements. Four patients had an improvement of 50% or more in their pain level. One patient measured 23% improvement in their pain level, while one patient 7% increase in pain level after the treatment. One patient measured 35% increased in pain level after the treatment because she miss understood on pain level questioner. The T-paired test score for before and after the treatment was 0.041707389, making the data gathered statistically irrelevant.

For the range of motion measurements there were small improvements on the averages of internal and external rotation of the shoulder both sides, arm length difference, and lateral bending to the left side. No change in the average of lateral bending to the right side, and decrease in Range of motion on forward flexion and extension of the neck. Only internal rotation of the left shoulder had a P-value of significance at 0.377138153. All other T-paired test values came as statistically irrelevant.

IV.   Conclusions from Neck and Shoulder Pain / Chronic study

VST acupuncture significantly improved neck and shoulder pain and provided improvement on ROM of the neck and shoulder areas. Also, VST acupuncture is effective in rebalancing of ROM and arm length differences in left and right side of body.

VST acupuncture contributes to provide protocols in diagnosis and systemized treatment for neck and shoulder pain and shows superior improvement of outcomes. It is recommended to perform future research with a large full-scale and long term period of treatment.

Korean

Kinetic

Acupuncture

Acupuncture's Next Generation

Muscle Trigger Point Technique

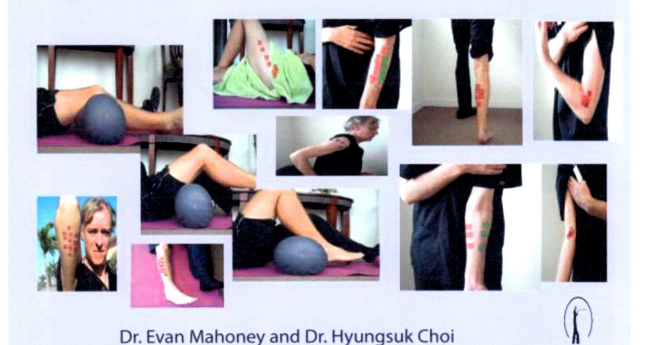

Dr. Evan Mahoney and Dr. Hyungsuk Choi

Korean Kinetic Acupuncture

Published by: Acupunctureandteas at www.acupunctureandteas.com

Please visit website for further information. Questions and comments can be sent to our blogsite www.evanmahoney.blogspot.com or at www.acupunctureandteas.com

Korean Kinetic Acupuncture: Acupuncture's Next Generation Muscle Trigger Point Technique

For the treatment of Pain and Pain Management

Table of Contents

Notes on the 2nd Edition

With pleasure I introduce the teachings of Dr. Hyungsuk Choi in this 2nd edition of Korean Kinetic Acupuncture. Dr. Choi is the creator of Kinetic Acupuncture and was my teacher/ mentor/ friend during my tenure at Samra Acupuncture Center's Doctoral program in Los Angeles, CA. It was the one of the greatest honors of my career to work so closely with and observe Dr. Choi's teachings and clinical practice.

He was a student /professor/ clinical practitioner at Kyunghee University, Korea. It is one of the most (if not the most) rigorous acupuncture schools in the world. From the grounds of this and other university experience Dr. Choi formulated the modern acupuncture technique of Kinetic Acupuncture. He continues to teach and lecture on this technique and is currently professor at Donkuk University in Los Angeles, CA.

Interjected in this 2nd edition are the notes and teachings direct from Dr. Choi's lectures and papers.

Dr. Hyungsuk Choi

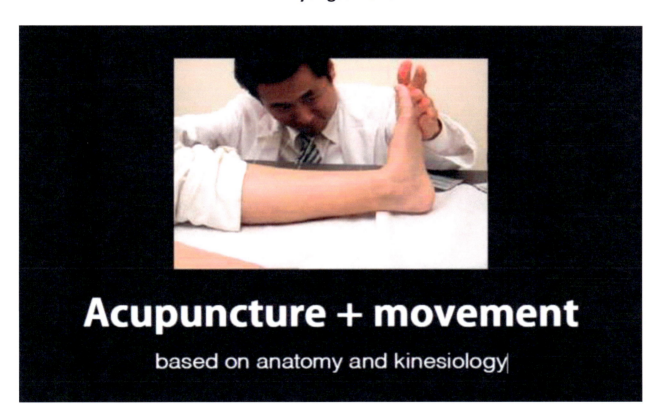

Our World Class Doctors Make the Difference.

Bringing the Best in Acupuncture to America

Samra clinics offer specialized acupuncture services, based upon years of scientific research and experience. Our physicians and specialists are leaders in their fields. The training of acupuncturists in Korea is quite rigorous, requiring ten years of academic study, internship, and residency. In fact, Korean Oriental medical schools are as selective and competitive to enter as conventional medical schools. Our doctors are at the top of their class and profession.

Key Seung Gwak, DC, LAc

(Professor of Oriental Medicine, Samra University)

- California Licensed Acupuncturist
- California Licensed Chiropractor
- NCCAOM Diplomate Acupuncture & Herbology
- D.C. Cleveland Chiropractic College
- Diplomate California Chiropractic Board
- Member of American Chiropractic Association
- Member of California Chiropractic Association
- Radiography Supervisor and Operator Permit, California

Hyungsuk Choi, CEO, PhD, LAc

(Professor of Oriental Medicine, Samra University)

- PhD, MS, Complementary and Alternative Medicine
  College of Medicine, Pochon CHA University
- B.A. Oriental Medicine, Kyung Hee University
- Researcher, Department of Herbology, Kyung Hee University
- Staff Physician (Oriental Medicine), Public Health Center
- Staff Physician (Oriental Medicine), Jangsu Oriental Medical Center
- Professional course of alternative medicine for cancer, Pochon CHA Univ. Graduate school of CAM
- Intern and Resident with Specialty of Acupuncture at Bosaeng, Oriental Medical Center
- Editor of Korean Oriental Association for Study of Obesity

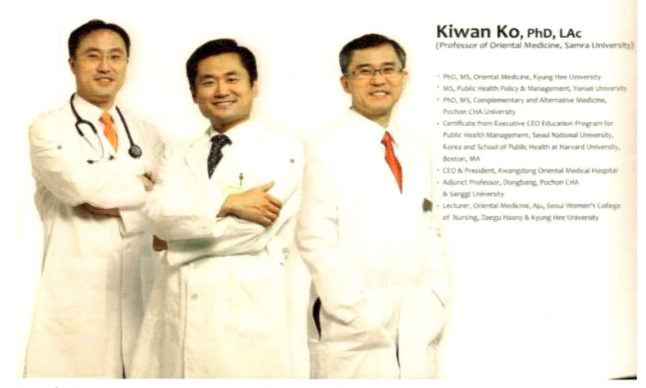

Kiwan Ko, PhD, LAc

(Professor of Oriental Medicine, Samra University)

- PhD, MS, Oriental Medicine, Kyung Hee University
- MS, Public Health Policy & Management, Yonsei University
- PhD, MS, Complementary and Alternative Medicine, Pochon CHA University
- Certificate from Executive CEO Education Program for Public Health Management, Seoul National University, Korea and School of Public Health at Harvard University, Boston, MA
- CEO & President, Kwangdong Oriental Medical Hospital
- Adjunct Professor, Dongbang, Pochon CHA & Sanggi University
- Lecturer, Oriental Medicine, Aju, Seoul Women's College of Nursing, Daegu Haany & Kyung Hee University

From the Samra Acupuncture Center Brochure printed in 2009

Inside Samra Acupuncture Center

At Samra Acupuncture Center, we take a 21st century approach to a 2000 year old discipline to p

Contemporary Diagnostic Tools

Unlike most acupuncture clinics which rely on questionnaires as their diagnostic tools, Samra Acupuncture Center utilizes state-of-the-art Magnetic Resonance Imaging (MRI), Nerve Conduction Velocity (NCV), and Digital X-Ray imaging to help us accurately pinpoint the origin of our patients' symptoms. We believe this is a crucial part of the acupuncture process, not only because it provides the clearest diagnoses, but it also rules out any life-threatening conditions which might require immediate medical intervention. At Samra Acupuncture Center, medical doctors, chiropractors and acupuncturists all work together, so that the patients' diagnoses and care are viewed from a comprehensive perspective.

Mobility + Acupuncture

"Keep your arms swinging, one-two, one-two, and one-two," leads the instructor as a young man performs what appears to be a formal and vigorous military march. This man is not in training for the army. He is being treated for back pain. If you look closely, you can see that he has barely visible acupuncture needles in his arms and legs. This is part of Samra Acupuncture Center's 'Mobility plus Acupuncture'. This unique treatment of needles and movement has helped alleviate severe and acute pain in many of our patients. Most patients experience immediate and extreme relief.

MRI Image

Our treatments deliver
- Pain relief
- Optimal function
- Balanced structure

Alignment

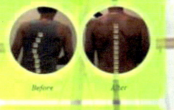

Before   *After*

Structure Balancing With Acupuncture

Structure + Function

Mobility

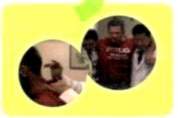

Passive & Active Exercise With Acupuncture

From Samra Brochure - Mobility Plus was the name given for Kinetic Acupuncture at the time

The Concept Behind
Möbility + Acupuncture

The body has both structure (**yin**) and function (**yang**); they are two sides of a coin. The human body should be treated as a whole, encompassing both aspects.

Structure

The human spine is like a mast on a sailboat. In order for the mast to be stable and upright, it must be sustained by many ropes. When we treat a patient's back pain, we do not work directly on the spine (**mast**), but rather on the muscles (**ropes**) attached to it. By using acupuncture, we can balance the tension of muscles and eventually obtain the proper stance of the spine.

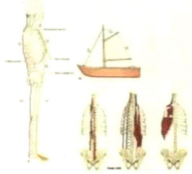

Function

In order to promote optimal function, we induce passive and active movements while needles are in place. Needles act to clear and dredge the blockages that can occur in muscles, joints or nerves. Active motion with needles in place improves the circulation of blood and oxygen to the area. This, in turn, helps to improve lubrication between tissues and promote healing.

Patients walk with needles or perform special workouts designed for their individual injury. In conventional acupuncture, the needles are inserted and the patient remains static. 'Mobility plus Acupuncture' treats the human body as a dynamic, moving entity.

Common Pains Treated by
Möbility + Acupuncture

The doctors at Samra Acupuncture Center use 'Mobility plus Acupuncture' for a wide variety of symptoms. In the treatment of lower back, shoulder, elbow, wrist or knee pain, the doctor will induce passive and active movements, while the needles are in place. This allows the doctor to stimulate the end of the joint cavity and all the muscles attached to the joint. Frozen shoulder patients who couldn't move their arms have been able to get dressed, lift their arms, and touch the opposite ear after just a few treatments.

At Samra Acupuncture Center, We Treat;

- **Spine related disorders**
  - Low back pain, neck pain, sciatica
  - Disc problems
  - Post surgical pain
- **Musculoskeletal pain**
  - Acute and chronic pain unresponsive to other treatments (Physical therapies, chiropractic care, epidural injections, etc.)
  - Doctors/ Patients want to explore a different approach
- **Workplace injuries (workers compensation)**
- **Personal injuries (traffic accidents)**
  - Treatment of unspecified pain
  - Restoration of function
- **Fibromyalgia**
- **Chronic fatigue syndrome**
- **Complex Regional Pain Syndrome**
- **Frozen shoulder / Impingement syndrome**
- **Knee complaints**

Covered by Major Insurance !

Call or Visit for Insurance verification
213-384-1100   www.samraclinic.com
1730 W. Olympic Blvd., Suite 100, Los Angeles, CA 90015

Samra Brochure - Written by Dr. Choi with assistance of Dr. Evan Mahoney

Acupuncture   Physio   Kinetics

Korean Kinetic Acupuncture

The following is from Dr. Hyungsuk Choi's lecture notes and slides on Kinetic Acupuncture.

Kinetic Acupuncture is one of the acupuncture techniques combined with movement, but several differences are there.

- KA has its own **unique principles** based on modern anatomy and kinesiology

- KA is Solution focused treatment

- Treatment session is **constant repeat of assessment and intervention** using treatment unit (acupuncture+movement)

KA Indication

Best for

Muscle originated Acute & Chronic Pain

- Lower Back Pain
- Muscle Sprain/ Strain, Spasm, Cramps
- Any joint or limb pain

-Motor weakness by nerve pathology
-Spinal injuries, foot drop

-Acute/ Chronic limited Range of Motion
-Frozen shoulder, aftermath of longterm
 immobilization

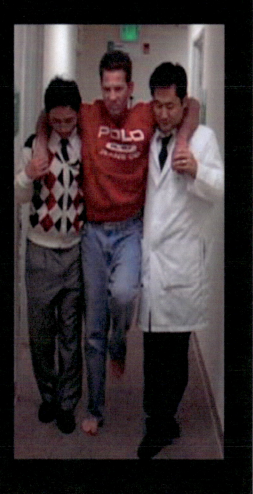

Movement to align spine to correct form. To strengthen and release back muscles.

Why movement?
- **We should treat (fix) moving things with movement (action).**
  "Healing is movement, disease is inertia" - Gabrielle Roth

- **Acupuncture helps movement by early pain control.**

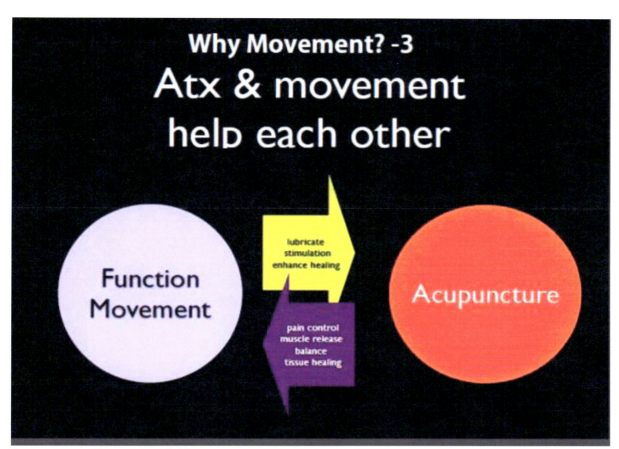

Acupuncture Treatment & Movement

Synergetic Effect: Atx & m

Stimulates Biological activity by moving synovial fluid, which brings nutrients to the avascular articular cartilage of the joint surfaces and intra-articular bibrocartilage of the minisci. Atrophy of

Both Atx and Movement help get more stimulus (blood flow) on acupoints and lubricate joints to help movement

(A) Real acupuncture

(B) Sham acupuncture

- More Blood flow means more nutrients and immune cells to tissue. Acupuncture can help remodel ligament, cartilage, and muscle.

- Kinetic Acupuncture helps muscles to stretch by removing trigger points

- Kinetic Acupuncture and movement balance whole body by adjusting muscle tone.

Kinetic acupuncture is Solution Focused Approach *

Kinetic Acupuncture is based on the belief that the patient heals themselves. By aiding proper functional recovery, acupuncture with movement accelerates the healing process. Therefore, the Kinetic Acupuncture practitioner focuses more on the solution than the etiology. Kinetic Acupuncture is not the process of getting rid of the cause, but the process of helping patient's healing.

The Kinetic Acupuncture practitioner applies the treatment unit, and sees the response, and intervenes again. Its depiction is like a conversation with the patient. Working closely with patient in active and passive exercise the Kinetic Acupuncture practitioner assesses and refines the needle placement and therapy based upon feedback from the patient and the physio kinetic response.   This is the foundation of the treatment plan triangle depicted later in the book.

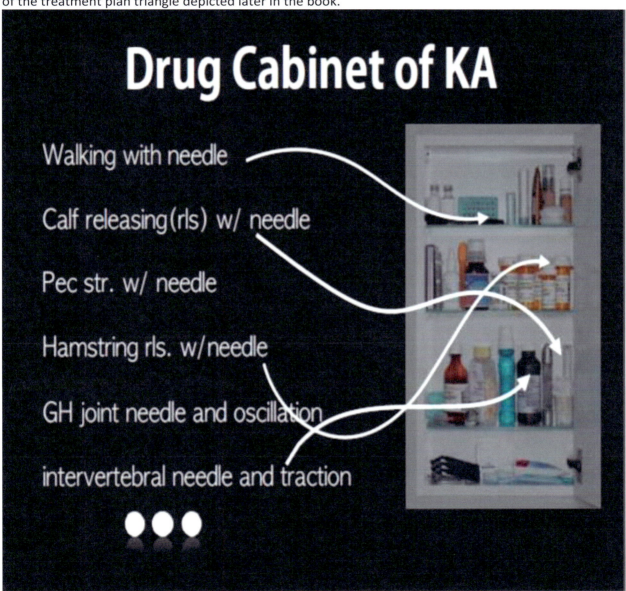

Different treatment units of Kinetic Acupuncture

*See additional commentary on Solution Focused Approach and the Prognosis Model - Appendix A

Three components of Kinetic Acupuncture

A. Joint cavity + joint play

Purpose - Aid local (connective tissue) healing by increased local blood flow, more immune cells and nutrient. Joint lubrication.

Indication - Frozen shoulder, knee pain, hip joint pain, back pain

Joint play - range of motion with kinetic acupuncture. Small amplitude motions of bones at joint surface. Traction, glide (or slide). Range of Motion exercises.

B. Muscle Trigger Points + Stretching & Strengthening

Purpose - Releasing or strengthening muscles for proper function

Indication - Motor weakness after stroke, spinal injury. Muscle tightness by overuse, bad posture. Balance problems with slackened or tightened muscles.

- Neck pain, back pain, hip joint pain, hemiplegia, foot drop, muscle soreness, bad posture, recurrent muscle spasm.

Technique - Trigger point on related muscle group.

Movement - isometric strengthening with needles, passive /active stretches with needles.

C. Traditional Acupuncture Points + functional coordination

Purpose - Enhance recovery of related muscles and coordination of antagonist synergistic muscles. Proprioception and mechanoreception stimulation.

Indication - All purpose indications. All kind of rehabilitation. Poor gait / balance, knee joint instability, "feeling of giving away."

Location - Distant and other acupuncture methods

Movements example - Walking with needles. Needle placement in points along the Large Intestine or Du channel while walking. Squat lunge, one legged squat lunge for balance.

Use of distant needles with complex movements.

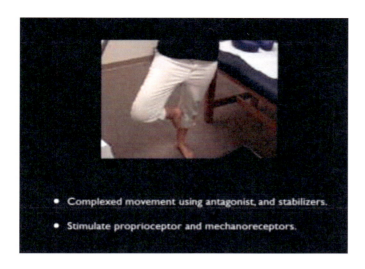

- Complexed movement using antagonist, and stabilizers.
- Stimulate proprioceptor and mechanoreceptors.

Kinetic Acupuncture is Solution Focused Approach

Example : ACL tear

We shifted our perspective from etiology to solution, so let's forget the ACL, and see what we can do for healing and moving

General pain control? Let's do tp on quad

Unbalance pelvis affect the load on knees? Gluteus tp and stretch

Prob with patella movement? joint cavity needle and joint play

for local(inside knee joint) healing? joint cavity and oscillation

One leg is loosing muscle tone? quad strengthening KA

Going back to work? track? Coordination, walking, balancing

*See additional commentary on Solution Focused Approach and the Prognosis Model - Appendix A

Introduction to Korean Kinetic Acupuncture by Dr. Evan Mahoney

Much of the groundwork for this book has been laid out in my previous books. Many of the stretches in the "Fountain of Youth" stretching series are derived from the Korean Kinetic Acupuncture Technique. The eight mechanisms of muscle trigger points and pathology explained in "Saam Korean Acupuncture: Advanced Combinations" and "VST Acupuncture: Capstone and Credentials" is also fundamental to the Korean Kinetic Acupuncture Technique.

I learned Korean Kinetic Acupuncture Technique from my teacher Dr. Hyungsuk Choi during my almost two year clinical residency and doctoral program at Samra Acupuncture Center. Samra Acupuncture Center was a busy pain management acupuncture clinic in the heart of Koreatown, Los Angeles. There we used Korean Kinetic Acupuncture, VST acupuncture, Saam Acupuncture and many other modalities for the treatment of pain. Dr. Choi is the creator of the Korean Kinetic Acupuncture technique.

The Korean Kinetic Acupuncture Technique; although modern, is part of the preeminent traditions of acupuncture and oriental medicine. They derive from acupuncture and were created by acupuncturist. These techniques should only be practiced by those properly and completely educated and clinically trained in the field of acupuncture and oriental medicine.

This book focuses on clinical applications for the treatment of pain, primarily pain of musculo - skeletal - tendon components. In general (barring tears or otherwise damaged muscles and tendons) pain of these types are a more favorable prognosis than pain of other structural natures such as spinal disc diseases, severe arthritis, or other tissue occlusion to joint cavities. The more severe structural diseases are usually a longer term development of what was an initial muscle tendon imbalance. In structural diseases there is often simultaneous musculo - skeletal - tendon imbalance which can make for a more favorable prognosis.

With the use of these techniques favorable results are often seen for general musculo -skeletal -tendon imbalance cases within the first treatment. The reader is encouraged to learn more about making a prognosis by reading "Choi Progression Analysis Chart" (see Appendix A). The ability to make a good prognosis is a skill which will give confidence in the face of your patients.

Do not hesitate to refer the patient out for a second opinion or to get an MRI, Xray, or other imaging study done if favorable results are not achieved within the first or second treatment and there still remains a mystery as to the diagnosis. This book will not explain musculoskeletal examination and diagnostic procedures and processes. The reader is encouraged to learn more about examination, diagnosis for pain if they are not already familiar. The practitioner should be familiar with red flag cases which need immediate referral out.

Further contraindications and safety from Dr. Choi.
Cautions in Case
-Active inflammatory or infected area
- Joint Ankylosis
-Avoid causing and increasing pain
-Any undiagnosed lesions
-Malignancy in the area
-Cauda equine lesions

These techniques are not limited to only pain but are also applied to tendon disorders such as trigger finger, hammer toe, and prevention of arthritic process and joint deformity.

Pain and the Eight Mechanisms of a Muscle Trigger Point (from "VST Acupuncture: Capstone and Credentials" and "Saam Korean Acupuncture: Advanced Combinations")

Trigger points are knots or nodules located in muscle tissue. The first mechanism that occurs due to the presence of knots in the muscle tissue is that the muscle becomes "SHORTENED". The analogy is if you take a piece of rope and tie it into a knot, it will shorten the length of that rope. Knots (Trigger Points) are clusters of fascia which tangle up and shorten the length of muscle.

The second mechanism that occurs due to trigger points is that they add increased tension and strain on the tendons. If the muscle is shortened it adds more strain on the tendon. A stretched and tightened tendon will likely rub with increased friction against adjacent tissues. Tendinitis (inflammation of the tendon) and muscle strains/ sprains are the most common injuries and diagnosis resulting from shortened muscles.

The third mechanism that occurs due to the presence of trigger points is the range of motion of the joint or limb will be decreased. The pull and strain from the shortened muscle and tightened tendon, simply will not allow the full range of motion of the joint or limb. When we do accidentally twist our foot or limb beyond its inhibited range of motion, a muscle sprain or strain will occur. Further damage such as a tear can also occur.

Fourth mechanism that occurs due to the presence of trigger points is that they inhibit the circulation of blood and oxygen to the muscle tissue. Blood and oxygen have a harder time circulating through the cluster of knotted tissue and fascia. The muscle becomes dehydrated. Dr. Hyungsuk Choi of Samra Acupuncture Center states the muscle tissue becomes a "Beef Jerky" like consistency, very dry and stringy.

Fifth Mechanism, a muscle that is dry and stringy with trigger points is unable to be strengthened. To strengthen, you must restore it to its normal length, tenderness, and pliability first.

Sixth Mechanism, the trigger point is painful upon palpation. The pain felt does not have to be local to the trigger point area. Pain will refer to points where the muscle attaches and inserts. Many painful diseases are actually located distantly away from where the trigger point occurs.

Seventh Mechanism is that trigger points can be present without any pain or physical complaint. Until a triggering event occurs (like accident, injury, or exposure to cold and ice). There may be no physical complaint even though the trigger point is present.

Eighth Mechanism: Peripheral Nerve Impingement. A shortened muscle/ stretched tendon may pinch on the nerves at the periphery (outside of the spinal column) causing radiating pain, numbness, or tingling down arms or joints. This is a more favorable prognosis as muscle stretching / tendon relaxation will eliminate the nerve impingement.

Cold

Muscle trigger points may lie dormant and be asymptomatic until a triggering event occurs such as an accident, muscle strain from heavy lifting, or falling. In acupuncture and oriental medicine cold is also a major factor behind the cause of pain. Much has been written of cold in my previous books and in regards to pain in "VST Acupuncture: Capstone and Credentials". The reader is encouraged to learn more of the mechanisms of cold and exposure points to cold from those books. In general cold triggers pain because it causes muscles to contract and blood vessels to constrict. This exasperates a muscle already shortened from trigger points and already restricted in blood circulation. In regards to taking a patient's history, when the cause of pain is a mystery and the onset is unclear, look to cold as the source and chief suspect.

Korean Acupuncture Techniques for the Treatment of Pain

VST (Vertex Synchronizing Technique) Acupuncture

VST acupuncture founded by Dr. Jonghwa Lee is a Korean Acupuncture Trigger Point Release Technique. VST acupuncture measures range of motion across the three planes (transverse, sagitall, coronal) of the neck, shoulder, lower back, and hip to identify affected antagonist muscles. VST then utilizes trigger point acupuncture to release the antagonistic muscle to restore range of motion and give pain relief. VST has applications across the entire body structures but for purposes of this paper VST will be used only for the vertexes of the neck/ shoulder, lower back and hips.

Agonist and Antagonist Muscles in VST and Korean Kinetic Acupuncture

Agonist Muscle: Muscle that initiates the action of movement of limb or body part.

Antagonist Muscle: Muscle that counters the action of agonist muscle, and creates movement of limb or body part counter to that of the agonist. In VST acupuncture the antagonist is identified as the shortened muscle causing the decrease in range of motion of joint or limb.

An example of the agonist / antagonist muscle is the biceps and triceps in flexion and extension of the forearm. To flex the forearm the biceps muscle initiates the movement. The biceps muscle contracts to move the forearm, it is the agonist muscle. While the biceps is contracting, the triceps extends and relaxes to allow the full movement of the joint or limb. The triceps muscle is the antagonist muscle when the forearm is flexing.

To extend the forearm the triceps muscle initiates the movement. The triceps contracts to straighten the forearm, it is the agonist muscle. As the forearm straightens, the biceps muscle extends and relaxes to allow the full movement. The biceps muscle is the antagonist muscle when the forearm extends.

In the antagonist role a muscle that is shortened will not allow for the full movement of joint or limb. In the above example if the biceps muscle is shortened due to the presence of knots, the full extension of the forearm will be limited. The patient will not be able to fully straighten their arm.

Korean Kinetic Acupuncture

Kinetic - pertaining to movement of joint, limb, neck, or torso. Korean Kinetic Acupuncture - Kinetic movement with Acupuncture. VST acupuncture is a muscle twitch trigger point release technique for the neck and lower back vertexes. Korean Kinetic Acupuncture is also a trigger point release technique. However it is not focused on achieving the "muscle twitch" response. Instead the trigger point is released through the isometric stretching exercises performed while the needles are in place. Korean Kinetic Acupuncture is performed upon the joints and limbs; the shoulders, elbows, wrist, feet, knee, and hips.

Isometric (Resistance) Stretching

For treatment of joints or limbs Isometric Stretching of targeted muscle may be the primary kinetic application with acupuncture. The targeted muscle will be stretched. In the stretched position the practitioner will add resistance as the muscle contracts to move the joint or limb. As the muscle contracts but is unable to move the joint or limb (due to resistance) the muscle will stretch. The needles remain inserted to the trigger points during the isometric stretch activity. The movement of the needle in the trigger point will facilitate a release and relaxation of the muscle, thereby achieving better range of motion and pain relief.

Caution: Never overstretch. Do not stretch beyond pain. Only stretch to the point that patient is comfortable with. Stretch to the point of muscle resistance, but not beyond.

Stretching is the answer

Much of the mechanisms of Muscle Trigger Point Pathology can be answered by stretching the muscle. With the activation of acupuncture, Korean Kinetic Acupuncture offers a superior way to stretch the muscles. The principles of acupuncture physiology offer a superior way for patients to remain in good health with pliable flexible muscles and overall general good health. Outside of the clinic the self stretching exercises in the "Fountain of Youth Stretching" series also offer a good way to remain pain free.

How this book works

Each chapter will explain the Korean Kinetic Acupuncture technique for the affected region of the body or disorder. In the clinic Korean Kinetic Acupuncture may be accompanied with other modalities and procedures. There is usually a certain order to the procedures being performed which defines the treatment plan. In general the first procedure for pain will either be VST or Korean Kinetic Acupuncture depending on the region of the body. A Treatment Plan Triangle will represent the order and procedure of techniques to be performed.

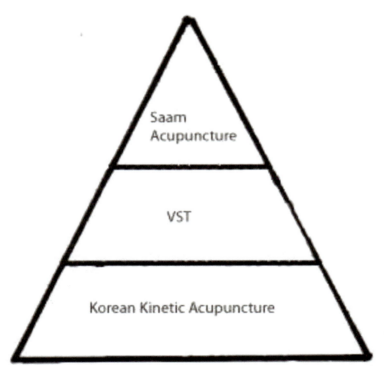

TREATMENT PLAN TRIANGLE

In this case the order of the procedure to be performed would be Korean Kinetic Acupuncture followed by VST acupuncture, followed by Saam Acupuncture. Korean Kinetic Acupuncture will always be performed as a separate procedure because it involves movement, exercise, and activity while the needles are in place. VST acupuncture can be used alone or combined at the same time as Saam Acupuncture (or whatever procedure the licensed acupuncturist prefers) because it is a passive technique used when the patient is stationary.

Mobilization and Kinetic Decompression Stretch are other procedures that may be included in the Treatment Plan Triangle. Other suggestions may fall outside of the triangle such as Moxibustion, Gua Sha muscle stretching or other techniques the practitioner has expertise in. These will be labeled as "Practitioners Choice" within the treatment plan triangle. There will also be self stretch recommendations for the patient to do at home based upon my "Fountain of Youth" muscle stretch series books. The practitioner will want to acquaint themselves with those materials as they provide integral insight and practice into these Korean Kinetic Acupuncture techniques.

Practitioner Choice

There are many branches of acupuncture and many specialized techniques. This book allows the practitioner to incorporate their specialized area of expertise with the techniques described herein.

Tuina Mobilization Techniques

Tuina Mobilization Techniques are vitally incorporated into VST and Korean Kinetic Acupuncture for the neck and lower back treatment.

There is one primary Tuina Mobilization Technique for Lower Back Pain. The Therapeutic Lumbar Technique (TLT) is used with every Lower Back Treatment. There are two components involved with (TLT). The first is a single Trigger Point Acupuncture insertion to the Quadratus Lumborum muscle. The needle is quickly inserted and quickly withdrawn. The needle is not retained. This technique will be demonstrated with its own chapter and video in the lower back section.

The other component of TLT is a back stretch which will not be demonstrated within these materials.

There are four primary Tuina Mobilization Techniques for the Neck. The Therapeutic Cervical Technique (TCT) is generally used with every Neck Treatment.

The components of TCT will not be demonstrated within these materials. Other than TCT #4.
TCT #4 is a simple acupressure technique at the suboccipital muscles. The patient is supine. The practitioner places the tips of their fingers (index,middle,ring) underneath Du 16, GB 20 as the patient relaxes their neck and head. Instructions to the patient are to take two deep inhalation/ exhalations and then relax. Hold the position for 1-2 minutes or longer per your wish. I will keep Saam Acupuncture needles in during this procedure, but I always remove any needles placed above the elbows, shoulders, neck and head. Never do TCT with needles in, above these areas.

This is the last of the four TCT components and is how we end our neck treatment.

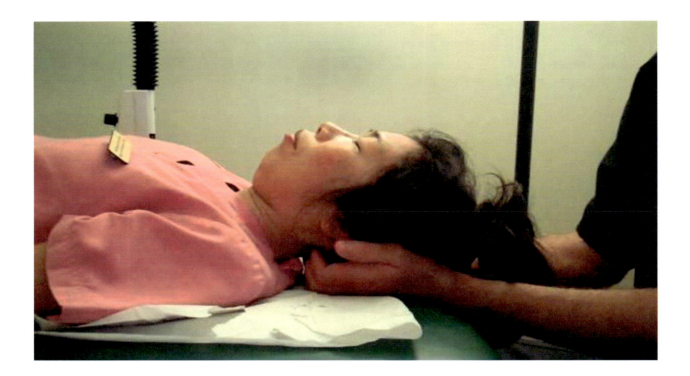

Video Demonstration

Attempts will be made to include a video demonstration of the Korean Kinetic Acupuncture procedures performed. The youtube link will be placed at the end of each chapter.

Cautions and Warnings

These techniques should only be performed by those licensed and educated in the full curriculum of acupuncture and oriental medicine. This includes completion of clinical education in a properly accredited acupuncture school. For purposes of this book these techniques should only be used for complaints of pain unless otherwise stated. It is to be understood that the practitioner using these techniques has a full understanding of acupuncture safety, contraindications, and proper needle location and insertion depth.

For purposes of Korean Kinetic Acupuncture the insertion depth of the needle will be no greater than .1-.3 cun unless otherwise stated. It is understood that the practitioner has a full understanding (western and eastern) of examination, diagnosis, disease conditions, illnesses, and structural injuries behind each of the pain conditions explained herein.

The practitioner using these techniques takes full responsibility for injuries or damages resulting from the use of said techniques. The author advises further clinical training for the practitioner before utilizing these techniques in the clinic.

Korean Kinetic Acupuncture for disorders of the hands, wrist, and fingers

Common disorders of the hand wrist and tendon - Tendonitis, pain, numbness, joint deformity, swelling, limited range of motion, Raynaud's syndrome.

In cases of numbness of the hands, wrists, and fingers or pain that radiates from the neck, shoulder, arm to the hands, wrist, and fingers, an extensive intake will have to be performed. The practitioner will have to determine if the cause is due to a central or peripheral nerve impingement syndrome. If it is of a central nerve impingement then there should be an accompanying complaint of neck/ shoulder pain or a history of neck injury or disease.

Red Flag - Radiating pain /numbness or bilateral radiating pain/ numbness, or if the patient is dropping objects held in hand then it is a likely a central nervous syndrome. Immediate referral to specialist for an MRI, Xray, or other imaging study is necessary. To be safe, if the patient has not been to another doctor, does not have a diagnosis, or has had no imaging studies done prior to seeing you, then refer out for further imaging study if no improvement is made after the first treatment.

Sometimes radiating pain or numbness is not of a series disorder. Alleviation of these symptoms may disappear after the use of these techniques. If so then the prognosis becomes more favorable.

For a simultaneous neck, shoulder, wrist complaint the practitioner will have to distinguish if there is a single event causing the symptoms or if there are simultaneous processes affecting each part individually. For instance numbness to the wrist or fingers can be a peripheral nerve impingement occurring at the forearm flexor / extensor muscles. This is usually due to repetitive over use of the hand and wrist in one's daily activities. It could be from a carpenter or laborer's use of a hammer or tool, too much time spent on the computer keyboard or mouse, or from a sports activity. Cold could be a factor too.

The patient may present with wrist, hand, or finger numbness along with a simultaneous neck /shoulder complaint. If so then a multitude of techniques could be implemented forming a treatment plan such as this.

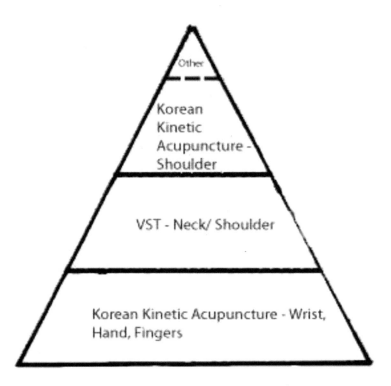

Wrist, Hand, Numbness with simultaneous Neck/ Shoulder complaint

In this treatment plan the practitioner will use the Korean Kinetic Acupuncture for the Wrist, Hands, and Fingers. The reason is to find out if the pain or numbness is alleviated after the use of the technique. If the pain or numbness recedes after the procedure has been performed then the diagnosis is much more favorable towards being only a local peripheral nerve impingement. In this case the Korean Kinetic Acupuncture Technique also becomes a diagnostic tool.

If no change to the numbness or hands has been made then the Korean Kinetic Acupuncture for the elbow can be performed. Essentially the practitioner works their way from distal to proximal of the neck and shoulder.

If the numbness has or has not receded after the Korean Kinetic procedures then VST can be performed for the neck and shoulder. Re-examine again. Maybe Korean Kinetic Acupuncture for the shoulder will be performed afterwards. Do moxibustion, mobilization, or other Practitioners Choice procedures. Re-examine the patient again. If there is still pain / numbness radiating to the wrist and hand then it should be recommended an MRI, Xray or other imaging study to find the diagnosis, if none has been made prior.

This example brings up some practical considerations for the Korean Kinetic Acupuncture procedures. These techniques may require more interaction with the patient. Thus more time spent with the patient. The techniques can be intensive and physically demanding. The practitioner is working in close proximity to the patient. The push and pull techniques of resistance stretching require strength and leverage of the entire body (especially during the Kinetic Shoulder procedure). Multiple procedures may be used.

Modification of treatment plans may be required depending upon the type of business model you have and the busyness of your clinic. Some patients may require multitude of procedures, other cases the problem will be resolved after a single kinetic procedure that only takes 5 or 10 minutes.

Sometimes we try to do too much for our patients, trying with one modality after the next to make an immediate difference. One can easily fall into this pattern because of the multitude of Korean Kinetic Acupuncture procedures and other techniques available.

Pain - Wrist, Hands, and Fingers

For general wrist, hand, finger complaints such as tendinitis with pain still in the acute -subacute time period, the prognosis is most favorable. Prior overuse may have been the cause. Cold too, should always be considered.

Korean Kinetic Acupuncture (KKA) should provide almost immediate relief and lasting benefits.

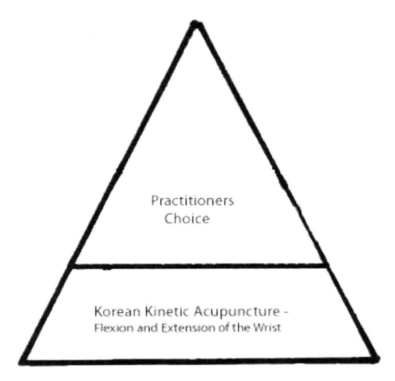

KKA - Extension and flexion of the wrist

Korean Kinetic Acupuncture Technique - Extension and Flexion of the Wrist.
To benefit the wrist, hands, and fingers.

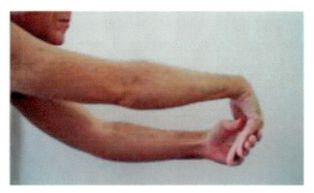

Wrist Flexion (right hand)
Normal wrist flexion 70-90 degrees

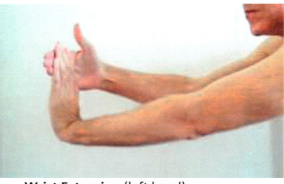

Wrist Extension (left hand)
Normal wrist extension is 65-85 degrees

The above pictures are the wrist and arm positions which we perform KKA in. The needles will have been inserted prior to extending or flexing the wrist.

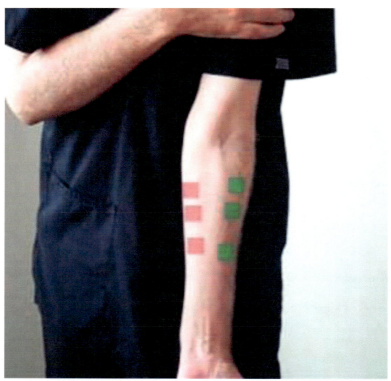

Anterior Forearm - Wrist Extension then Flexion - KKA Targeted Muscles

The main wrist flexor muscles targeted with Korean Kinetic Acupuncture are Flexor Carpi Radialis, Palmaris Longus, and Flexor Carpi Ulnaris (highlighted in pink in the photograph). The Brachioradialis (highlighted in green) is not a wrist flexor but is a muscle you may want to target with KKA.

Shortened muscles cause imbalance along the chain

By stretching the wrist flexors we can also accomplish stretching and releasing of the smaller flexor muscles of the hands and fingers.

When the wrist flexors are shortened, more tension is added to the attaching tendons. This causes joint mal-alignment as well as additional tension to attached tendons and muscles further along the chain of the structure. In doing Korean Kinetic Acupuncture for wrist flexion we will also be affecting the hand and finger flexors as well. So a benefit to the whole hand can be derived from this procedure.

KKA Wrist Flexion - The Procedure

Wrist flexion is the action taken, while the wrist is in extended position.

Done in the seated position with practitioner and patient facing one another.

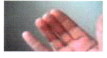

1. Find the trigger point, knotted areas of the wrist flexors.
- Extend the patients hand (which stretches the flexors). In the stretched position, the practitioner massages in a distal to proximal direction with the three middle fingers firmly pressed against the patient's anterior forearm.

2. Insert needles into trigger point areas of wrist flexors (superficial .1-.3 cun). The patients hand is not stretched; neither flexed, nor extended during insertion of needles.

3. Test patient comfort level with needles by moving the hand back and forth between flexion and extension. Adjust the needle outward if discomfort. Watch for dimples surrounding the needle insertion area during movement. Dimple areas may indicate discomfort, adjust the needle outward.

4. Patient comfort with the needles has been assured with a test movement of the wrist.

Begin Isometric Resistance

The patients elbow is kept straight throughout the procedure. The practitioner can use one hand (if necessary) to support the straightened elbow.

The practitioner gently brings the patients wrist and hand as far as comfortable in the extended position. (In the seated position with practitioner facing patient, the patients arm is supine with fingers pointed towards the floor, during extension of the wrist.) With the wrist in full extended stretch, the patient is instructed to flex the wrist and hand against the resistance of the practitioner's hand (which is placed across the patient's palmer area).

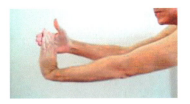

In the wrist extension picture above, the practitioner assumes the role of the right hand as it resists the patients attempt to flex their hand.

To the practitioner's count of four the patient flexes their hand against the resistance of the practitioner. At "four" the patient is instructed to "relax". The practitioner returns the hand again to extended stretch as far as patient is comfortable.

The exercise is repeated 5- 10 times. Remove the needles immediately upon the last isometric resistance stretch.

Added variation for finger complaints (trigger finger, joint pain, etc).
If patient has a finger complaint you would still begin with the wrist flexion procedure described above. With needles retained extend the hands and fingers as far as patient is comfortable with. The practitioner will be holding and resisting the patient's fingers. Ask the patient to flex their fingers against the resistance of the practitioner's hand. This can be done individually upon each of the fingers.

KKA Wrist Extension

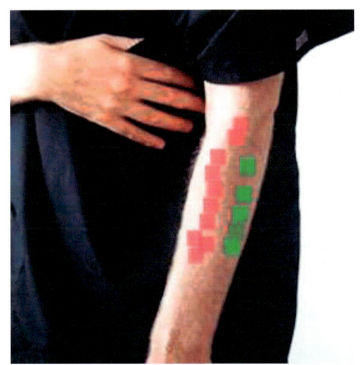

Posterior Forearm - Wrist Extension - KKA Targeted Muscles

The main wrist extensor muscles targeted with Korean Kinetic Acupuncture are Extensor Carpi Radialis Longus, Extensor Carpi Radialis Brevis, Extensor Digitorum Communis (highlighted in pink in the photograph). Extensor Carpi Ulnaris (highlighted in green).

This procedure can help conditions at the elbow such as Tennis Elbow affecting the Lateral Epicondyle of the humerus which is the attachment point for Extensor Carpi Radialis Brevis. Use in combination with the KKA - Elbow procedure.

KKA Wrist Extension - The Procedure
Done in the seated position with practitioner and patient facing one another.

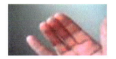

1. **Find the trigger point, knotted areas of the wrist extensors.**
- Flex the patient's hand (which stretches the extensors). Done in the position demonstrated in the picture below. In the stretched position, the practitioner massages in a distal to proximal direction with the three middle fingers firmly pressed against the patient's posterior forearm.

2. Insert needles into trigger point areas of wrist extensors (superficial .1-.3 cun). The patients hand is not stretched; neither flexed, nor extended during insertion of needles.

3. Test patient comfort level with needles by moving the hand back and forth between flexion and extension. Adjust the needle outward if discomfort. Watch for dimples surrounding the needle insertion area during movement. Dimple areas may indicate discomfort, adjust the needle outward.

4. Patient comfort with the needles has been assured with a test movement of the wrist.

Begin Isometric Resistance

The patients elbow is kept straight throughout the procedure. The practitioner can use one hand (if necessary) to support the straightened elbow.

The practitioner gently brings the patients wrist and hand as far as comfortable in the flexed position. With the wrist in full flexed stretch, the patient is instructed to extend the wrist and hand against the resistance of the practitioner's hand (which is placed across the patient's dorsal area of hand).

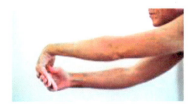

In the wrist flexion picture above, the practitioner assumes the role of the right hand as it resists the patients attempt to extend their hand. To the practitioner's count of four the patient extends their hand against the resistance of the practitioner. At "four" the patient is instructed to "relax". The practitioner returns the hand again to flexed stretch as far as patient is comfortable.

The exercise is repeated 5- 10 times. Remove the needles immediately upon the last isometric resistance stretch.

Assess the patient after the flexion / extension procedures are finished.

 Ask them if they feel a difference. Ask them to move their wrist and arms, curl their fingers. They should have improved range of motion, less pain. Maybe a trigger finger is able to return to position more smoothly?

If a difference has been made, it is a most favorable prognosis. Likely the result of musculo - tendon imbalance.

After Korean Kinetic Acupuncture for both wrist extension and flexion has been completed, practitioner has their choice as to how else treat the condition.

Video Demonstration of Wrist Extension/ Flexion exercises

https://www.youtube.com/watch?v=iRwdB-fp7fc

Elbow Lateral Side

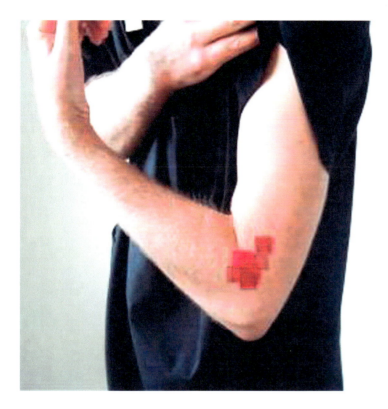

The Brachialis and Brachioradialis are major targeted muscles for conditions affecting the lateral elbow. The Brachialis flexes the forearm, the Brachioradialis supinates the forearm.   A primary complaint might be Tennis Elbow, which is also treated using the **KKA Wrist Extension Procedure**.

KKA Procedure Elbow Lateral Side
Done in the seated position with practitioner and patient facing one another.

The patients arm will be pronated and slightly flexed upon a cushion sitting atop either the lap of the practitioner or patient. This is the stretched position for the Brachialis and Brachioradialis.

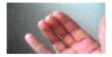

1. **Find the trigger point, knotted areas around the elbow.**
- Massage in a distal to proximal direction with the three middle fingers firmly pressed against the patient's lateral elbow.

2. Insert needles into trigger point areas of Brachialis and Brachioradialis (Acupoint Large Intestine 11 and surrounding area. **Superficial .1-.3 cun).** The patients arm is relaxed upon a cushion on the practitioner (or patient's) lap.

3. Test patient comfort level with needles by moving the arm and elbow in a motion mimicking the backhand swing in Tennis (Flexion and Supination of forearm). Adjust the needle outward if discomfort. Watch for dimples surrounding the needle insertion area during movement. Dimple areas may indicate discomfort, adjust the needle outward.

4. Patient comfort with the needles has been assured with a test movement of the elbow.

Begin Isometric Resistance

Mimicking the movement of a backhand swing in tennis, the practitioner adds resistance across the back of the hand and arm as the patient tries to both flex and supinate the forearm.

To the practitioner's count of four the patient tries to lift their forearm against the resistance of the practitioner. At "four" the patient is instructed to "relax". The practitioner returns the arm again to resting position upon the cushion.

The exercise is repeated 5- 10 times. Remove the needles immediately upon the last isometric resistance stretch.

Elbow Medial Side

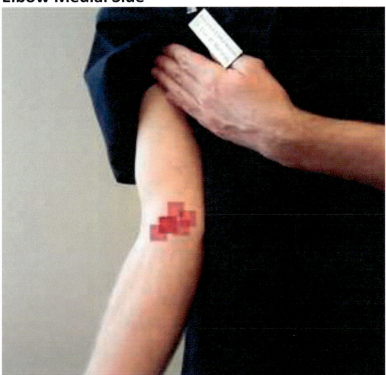

The Pronator Teres is the primary muscle affecting the medial elbow. A primary complaint might be Golfers Elbow which affects the Pronator Teres and Flexor Carpi Radialis and Ulnaris (which were treated using **KKA Wrist Flexion Procedure**.

KKA Procedure Elbow Lateral Side

Done in the seated position with practitioner and patient facing one another.

The patients arm will be supinated and extended upon a cushion sitting atop the lap of either the practitioner or patient. This is the stretched position of the Pronator Teres.

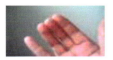

1. **Find the trigger point, knotted areas around the elbow.**
- Massage in a distal to proximal direction with the three middle fingers firmly pressed against the patient's medial elbow.

2. Insert needles into trigger point areas of Pronator Teres (Acupoint Heart 3 **superficial .1-.3 cun).** The patients arm is relaxed upon a cushion on the practitioner (or patient's) lap.

3. Test patient comfort level with needles by moving the arm and elbow in a motion mimicking the motion of an arm wrestler (Flexion and pronation of forearm). Adjust the needle outward if discomfort. Watch for dimples surrounding the needle insertion area during movement. Dimple areas may indicate discomfort, adjust the needle outward.

4. Patient comfort with the needles has been assured with a test movement of the elbow.

Begin Isometric Resistance

Mimicking the movement of an arm wrestler, the practitioner adds resistance across the palmer hand wrist area as the patient tries to both flex and pronate the forearm.

To the practitioner's count of four the patient tries to lift their forearm against the resistance of the practitioner. At "four" the patient is instructed to "relax". The practitioner returns the arm again to resting position upon the cushion.

The exercise is repeated 5- 10 times. Remove the needles immediately upon the last isometric resistance stretch.

Tennis Elbow - Treatment Plan Triangle

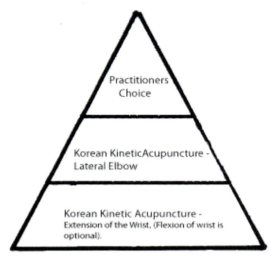

Practitioners Choice

Korean KineticAcupuncture - Lateral Elbow

Korean Kinetic Acupuncture - Extension of the Wrist, (Flexion of wrist is optional).

Flexion of the Wrist is optional but Recommended

Golfers Elbow - Treatment Plan Triangle

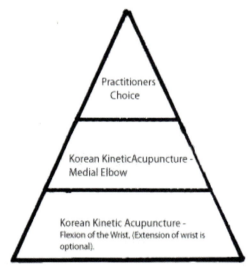

Practitioners Choice

Korean KineticAcupuncture - Medial Elbow

Korean Kinetic Acupuncture - Flexion of the Wrist, (Extension of wrist is optional).

Extension of wrist is optional but Recommended

Video Demonstration of Elbow Medial / Lateral

https://www.youtube.com/watch?v=INBsq81-sOk

Triceps and Elbow - Inability to Fully Flex the Arm

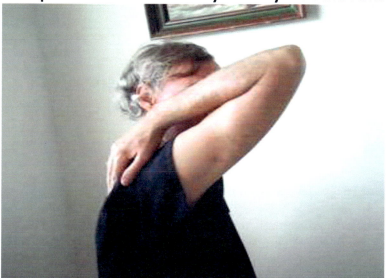

Normal elbow flexion 150 degrees - the forearm should touch biceps

The inability to fully flex the elbow or pain at the posterior aspects of the elbow may be a result of muscle shortening in the Triceps area.   In the picture above the forearm is flexed. The biceps are the agonist muscle (initiating flexion) while the triceps are the antagonist inhibiting the action. With shortened triceps due to muscle trigger points there will be loss of range of motion and pain.

KKA Procedure Triceps and Elbow

The picture above is exactly the position which the practitioner will want to insert the needles into the patient. Both the Shoulder and the forearm are flexed.

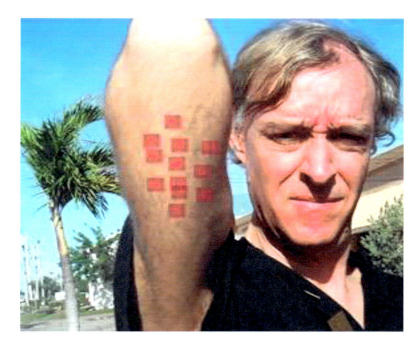

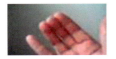

Starting in the forearm and shoulder fully flexed position (the triceps is fully stretched).

1. Find the trigger point, knotted areas on the Triceps.
- Massage in a distal to proximal direction (from elbow to shoulder) with the three middle fingers firmly pressed against the patient's triceps.

2. Insert needles into trigger point areas of Triceps (superficial .1-.3 cun).

3. Test patient comfort level with needles by moving the patient's forearm in extension and flexion direction. (Keep the shoulder flexed). Adjust the needle outward if discomfort. Watch for dimples surrounding the needle insertion area during movement. Dimple areas may indicate discomfort, adjust the needle outward.

4. Patient comfort with the needles has been assured with a test movement of the forearm.

Begin Isometric Resistance
Starting in the forearm and shoulder fully flexed position. The practitioner instructs the patient to extend their forearm against the resistance of the practitioner (practitioner's resisting hand is placed proximal to patients wrist).

To the practitioner's count of four the patient tries to extend their forearm against the resistance of the practitioner. At "four" the patient is instructed to "relax". The practitioner returns the forearm to the flexed position as far as the patient is comfortable with.

The exercise is repeated 5- 10 times. Remove the needles immediately upon the last isometric resistance stretch.

Video Demonstration of Triceps Procedure

https://www.youtube.com/watch?v=woCs0el9Zk8

Shoulder

The Korean Kinetic Acupuncture Procedure for the Shoulder does not specifically target muscle trigger points or specific muscles of the shoulder. This is because the companion technique VST (Vertex Synchronizing Technique) Acupuncture does provide for trigger point release of the four shoulder rotator cuff muscles, deltoid, and neck muscles.

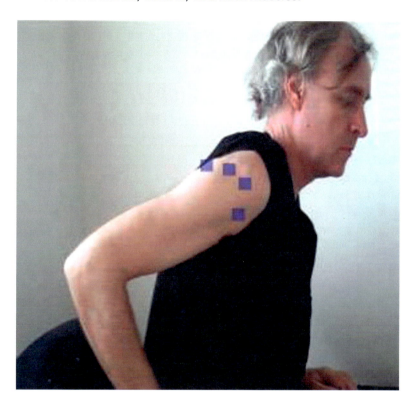

The KKA procedure for the shoulder is the secondary procedure to VST neck. It uses a combination (practitioners choice) of traditional acupuncture points San Jiao 14, Large Intestine 15, Small Intestine 9,10, and extra point Jianqian with shoulder movement and isometric resistance. Usually only three points are chosen, LI 15, SJ 14, and Jianqian.

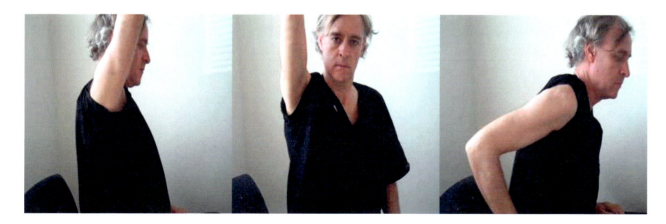

Normal shoulder flexion 180 degrees.   Normal Shoulder extension between 45-60 degrees

KKA Procedure Shoulder

1. Insert needles into the acupuncture points Large Intestine 15, San Jiao 14, and Jianqian (superficial .1-.3 cun).

2. Test patient comfort level with needles by moving the patient's shoulder in extension and flexion direction. (Patient should keep their shoulder relaxed). Adjust the needle outward if discomfort. Watch for dimples surrounding the needle insertion area during movement. Dimple areas may indicate discomfort, adjust the needle outward.

3. Patient comfort with the needles has been assured with a test movement of the shoulder.

Kinetic Movement #1 for Shoulder

The practitioner holding the patient at the wrist and supporting at the shoulder, gently rocks the arm and shoulder in a lateral and medial direction at the same time as moving the shoulder in flexion/ extension, up and down (no greater than 90 degrees in flexion, 50 degrees in extension).   The gentle rocking motion in the lateral / medial plane can be achieved by the practitioners grip at the wrist.

Kinetic Movement #2 Begin Isometric Resistance

The practitioner passively flexes the patients shoulder to 180 degrees or as far as the patient is comfortably able to go. Practitioner then instructs the patient to extend and adduct their shoulder "pull down" against resistance of the practitioner. The practitioner's resisting hand is placed underneath the patients elbow.

To the practitioner's count of four the patient tries to "pull down", adduct and extend their shoulder against the resistance of the practitioner. At "four" the patient is instructed to "relax". The practitioner returns the shoulder to the flexed position as far as the patient is comfortable with.

The exercise is repeated 5- 10 times. The shoulder is gently assisted to resting posture by the practitioner. Remove the needles immediately upon the last isometric resistance.

Treatment Plan Triangle Shoulder

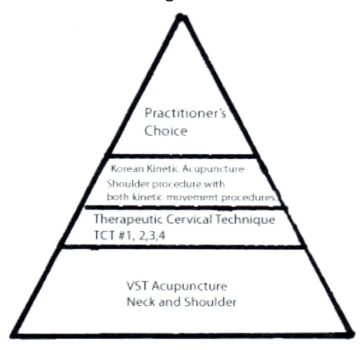

Practitioner's Choice

Korean Kinetic Acupuncture Shoulder procedure with both kinetic movement procedures.

Therapeutic Cervical Technique TCT #1, 2,3,4

VST Acupuncture Neck and Shoulder

Video Demonstration of Shoulder KKA technique

https://www.youtube.com/watch?v=AYwMS_bKhcM&feature=youtu.be

Plantar Foot / Heel Problems - Root of problem is Calf Muscle (Gastrocnemius) Shortening.

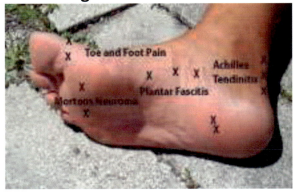

Following is an excerpt from my book "Dr. Evan Mahoney's Fountain of Youth Stretching"

Calf Muscle Stretch - for Plantar Fascitis, Achilles Tendinitis, Mortons Neuroma

The Calf Muscle Stretch is a great stretch for the feet, especially for pain relief from Plantar Fasciitis, Morton's Neuroma, and Achilles Tendinitis. Even though these pain conditions are located on the bottom of the foot or at the heel, the true root and core of the problem lies in the calf muscle.

Due to postural imbalance, wearing high heels, and not stretching; the calf muscles will develop knots which shorten and contract the muscles. Because the muscles are shortened there is added tension upon the Achilles tendon, which attaches to underlying tendons and carriage of the foot. The increase of tension upon the tendons causes rubbing and friction against adjacent tissues which leads to tendonitis, calcification deposits, and neuromas. Because of the uneven tension of the muscles and tendons the alignment of joints is likely to be pulled out of balance.

We stretch the muscle to relax the tension upon the tendons.

Fountain of Youth Calf Muscle Stretch Technique
The calf muscle stretch I perform is a variation off of the common calf muscle stretch.
In doing this stretch bring the foot back as far as possible so that the heel of the foot is still touching the ground.

Next, push against the wall with your hands. As you push against the wall with the hands this will help to drive the heel into the ground, which provides a greater degree of stretch for the calf.

Hold the stretch for 20 seconds take a break and then repeat.

If there is any pain or discomfort doing this stretch then pull off and take a break.

Place the foot back is as far as possible so the heel is still touching the ground. Push against the wall with hands. This will drive downward force of the heel into the ground, further accentuating Calf Muscle Stretch. Hold for 20 Seconds.

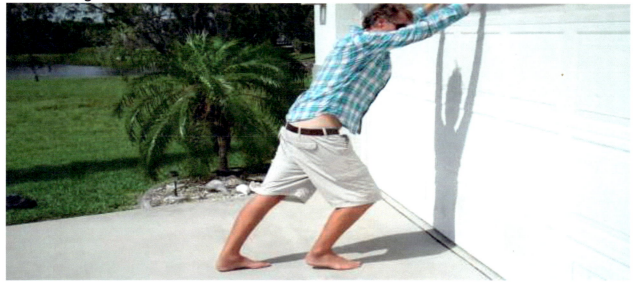

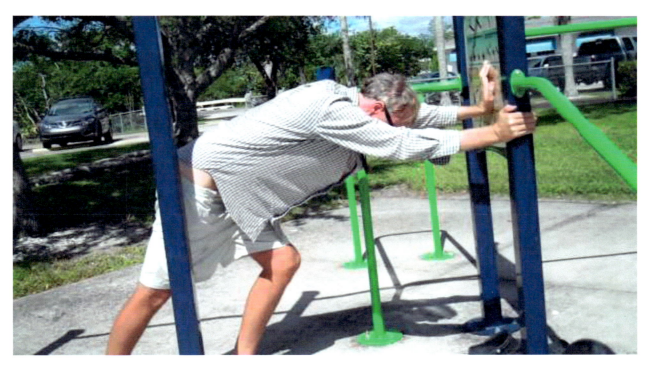

Arms and hands may be placed low upon the wall or object in order to draw heel back as far as possible.

KKA Calf Muscle Stretch- The Procedure

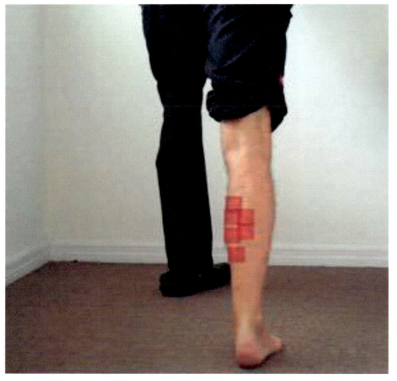

There are two components to the Korean Kinetic Acupuncture Procedure for releasing Muscle Trigger Points along the calf and stretching the muscle.

Procedure 1 - Is an Isometric Resistance exercise.

Procedure 2 - Is a repeat of the stretch technique described above.

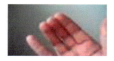

Start with the patient standing in the calf muscle stretch position. The patient's foot is placed as far back as possible so the heel is still touching the ground. The practitioner will be sitting upon the ground near the patient's foot and heel.

1. Find the trigger point, knotted areas on the Calf Muscle. In almost all cases the muscle trigger points will be located on the Medial Gastrocnemius (pictured above).

- Massage in a distal to proximal direction (from heel to knee) with the three middle fingers firmly pressed against the patient's medial calf muscle.

2. Insert needles into trigger point areas of Medial Gastrocnemius Muscle (superficial .1-.3 cun).

3**. Test patient comfort level with needles by asking them to stand up and down on their toes, lifting the heel off the ground, keeping the toes on the ground. This is a <u>Foot and Ankle Plantar Flexion exercise</u>, the Gastrocnemius contracts to lift the heel off the ground**. Adjust the needles outward if discomfort. Watch for dimples surrounding the needle insertion area during movement. Dimple areas may indicate discomfort, adjust the needle outward.

4. Patient comfort with the needles has been assured with a test movement of the foot.
Caution: Make sure the patient does not feel dizzy, lightheaded, or feint, during the massage palpation and needle insertion phase. Oftentimes the patient is unaware of the painful trigger point areas on the calf muscle. Even palpation alone can sometimes cause them to feel dizzy or feint. At all times during the procedure, communicate and assure them of their comfort level. Prepare yourself in case they should fall.

In another sense it is assuring to have pain upon palpation at the muscle trigger points. If there is the presence of knots and tenderness upon palpation the practitioner will be much more assured of their diagnosis and prognosis. The diagnosis is the knots at the calf muscle are the root of the problem and not at the painful area of the foot. The prognosis is favorable with the Korean Kinetic Acupuncture technique.

Begin Isometric Resistance

Procedure 1 - Resistance against the Foot and Ankle Plantar Flexion exercise.
With needles in place the patient is in the fully stretched Calf Muscle Stretch position (heel touching the ground). The practitioner instructs the patient to lift their heel off the ground against the resistance of the practitioner (practitioner's hand is gripped at the posterior ankle and heel). As the patient lifts their foot off the ground, the practitioner can actively push down against this motion as they grip at the ankle. **Caution: sometimes the grip itself (not the needles) can cause the patient pain. If so modify the grip with less resistance.**

To the practitioner's count of four the patient will lift their heel off the ground against the resistance of the practitioner. At "four" the patient is instructed to "relax". The patient returns their foot and heel to the floor.

The exercise is repeated 5- 10 times. Remove the needles immediately upon the last isometric resistance stretch.

*The practitioner will get a sense of the physical strength required to perform certain Kinetic procedures like this.

Procedure 2*
After Procedure 1 has been performed the practitioner instructs the patient to move their heel back (needles still in place on Gastrocnemius) even farther. As far back as the foot will go, so the heel still

touches the ground. The patient will then be instructed to perform the stretch technique described above.

With arms against the wall, the patient will "push" into the wall. This force will pass through the body and will drive the heel into the ground, further stretching the calf muscle. The patient will hold for 20 seconds, as the practitioner counts off. The practitioner may also want to accentuate this stretch by gripping at the ankle and pushing the heel into the ground.

Repeat Procedure 1 again

With the foot still in the same far back position (heel touching the ground) repeat Procedure 1 again, one more time after Procedure 2.

Variation of Procedure 2 - specific for Mortons Neuroma

Mortons Neuroma is a painful condition usually affecting the bottom of the third or fourth toe at the ball of the feet. A nodule may be present that feels to the patient like they are standing on a pebble. According to the second principle of Muscle Trigger points (mentioned in the opening chapter) friction occurs as stretched tendons rub against adjacent tissue. This can lead to calcification and the development of nodules.

Mortons Neuroma can be a latter development of shortened calf muscles, which adds tension upon the Achilles tendon, which adds tension to the tendons on the undercarriage of the foot.

Variation of Procedure 2 is as follows.

As the patient is pushing against the wall in the calf muscle stretch position (heel touching the ground), the practitioner reaches under the toes and lifts them up (extending them). The toes can be extended to the practitioners count of "four" and then relax. Repeat this exercise during the duration of the 20 second stretch that the patient is in.

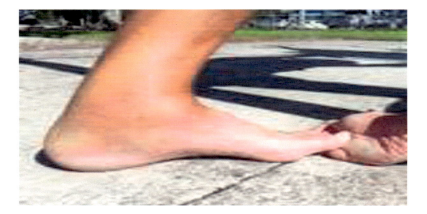

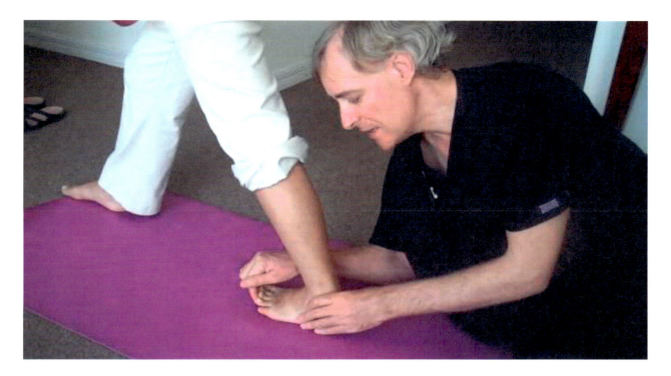

These are examples of lifting the toes up during the calf muscle stretch, as part of variation to Procedure #2. Lift, count to 4, relax.

*Procedure 2 is my creation, which is a variation off of Procedure 1 which I learned from Dr. Choi.

Treatment Plan Triangle for pain, conditions affecting heel, plantar aspect of the foot.

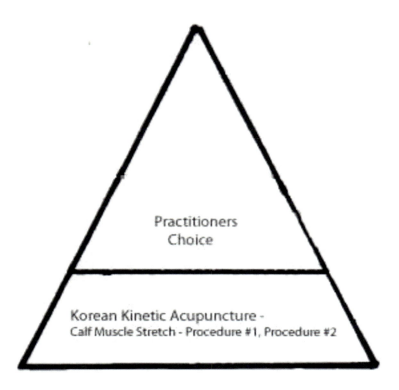

Video Demonstration of Calf Muscle Stretch for Plantar Fascitis

https://www.youtube.com/watch?v=IiWNqRtV6n0

Dorsal Foot / Toe Problems - Root of problem is Anterior Tibialis Muscle Shortening.

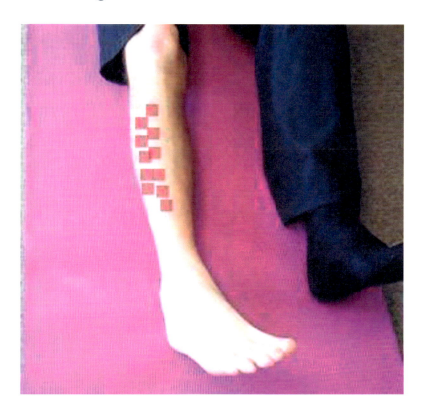

The primary muscles for this KKA procedure are the Anterior Tibialis and Extensor Digitorum Longus which contract to dorsi flex the foot and extend the toes. Common problems may be tendinitis along the dorsum of the foot and toe malformation like hammer toe. These can be a result of muscle shortening, adding tension to the tendons along the muscle tendon chain of the foot and toes.

There are also two procedures for muscle trigger point release of the Anterior Tibialis and Extensor Digitorum Longus. The first is KKA with needles and the second is a stretch only without needles.

Procedure 1 - KKA with Isometric Resistance

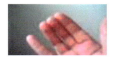

Patient is lying supine on the table with foot and leg stretch (as in picture above). There is no cushion under the knee, the leg is kept straight. The practitioner presses down on the top of foot and toes to Dorsi Flex the foot. In the Dorsiflex position the Anterior Tibialis is stretched.

1. Find the trigger point, knotted areas on the Anterior Tibialis.

- Massage in a distal to proximal direction (from ankle to knee) with the three middle fingers firmly pressed against the patient's Anterior Tibialis.

2. Insert needles into trigger point areas of Anterior Tibialis (acupoints anywhere along Stomach 36-40 and Gall Bladder 34 - 39) (superficial .1-.3 cun).

3. Test patient comfort level with needles by moving the patient's foot in extension and flexion direction. (Keep the leg straight). Adjust the needle outward if discomfort. Watch for dimples surrounding the needle insertion area during movement. Dimple areas may indicate discomfort, adjust the needle outward.

4. Patient comfort with the needles has been assured with a test movement of the foot.

Begin Isometric Resistance

Starting in the leg straight and foot plantar flexed position (the Anterior Tibialis is stretched). The practitioner instructs the patient to extend their foot upwards against the resistance of the practitioner (practitioner's resisting hand is placed atop the dorsal aspect of the patient's foot).

To the practitioner's count of four the patient tries to extend their foot against the resistance of the practitioner. At "four" the patient is instructed to "relax". The practitioner returns the foot to the plantar flexed position as far as the patient is comfortable with.

The exercise is repeated 5- 10 times. Remove the needles immediately upon the last isometric resistance stretch.

Procedure 2 - KKA stretch only

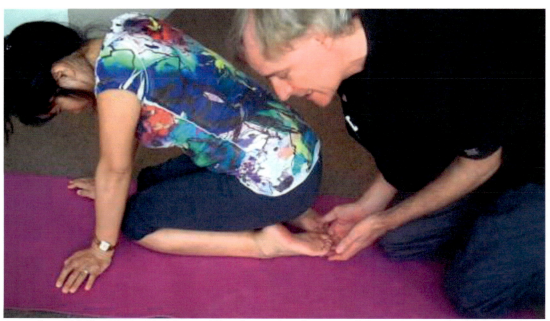

Anterior Tibialis. The practitioner lifts the patient's toes while Anterior Tibialis is stretched. Practitioner counts to 4 and then relaxes the stretch (returning toes to ground). Repeat 5-10 times.

Anterior Tibialis Stretch (excerpt taken from "Fountain of Youth Stretching")

Caution: The knees may prohibit the ability to sit completely upon ones legs. Do not force yourself (or the patient) if there is pain or resistance at the knees. If there is difficulty in doing this stretch because of the knees then do the knee stretch (described in a later chapter) before doing the anterior tibialis stretch.

If there is pain at the top of the foot doing this stretch, stop the stretch and relax. The muscles and tendons may be too tight in the beginning and the potential to over stretch, strain, sprain or tear the muscle or tendon is possible.

Fountain of Youth Anterior Tibialis Stretching Technique

To stretch the Anterior Tibialis Muscle, sit upon your knees. Sit firmly so the butt is pressing on the back of the legs and heels. From this position, reach under the toes and lift them off the ground.

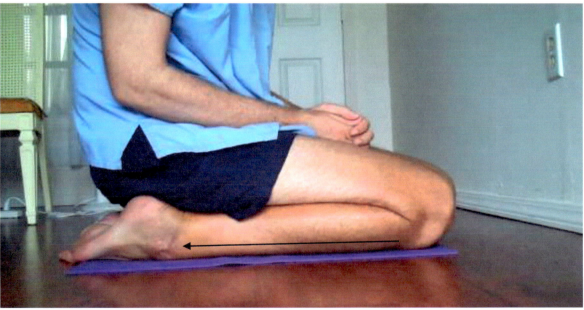

Anterior Tibialis in a Stretch

To further stretch the Anterior Tibialis reach under your toes (one foot at a time) count to four and then release.

In Procedure 2 for KKA Anterior Tibialis Stretch - the practitioner will lift the toes up for the patient. Hold for the count of "4" then "relax", repeat lifting the toes, count to "4" then "relax". Repeat 5-10 times.

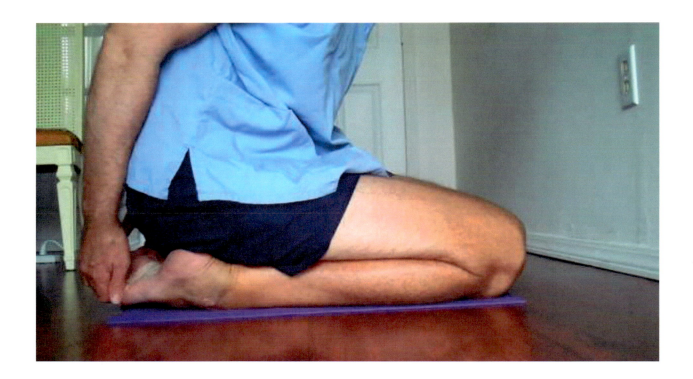

Treatment Plan Triangle for pain, conditions affecting dorsi aspect of the foot.

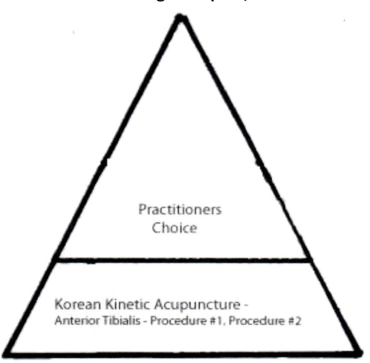

Practitioners
Choice

Korean Kinetic Acupuncture -
Anterior Tibialis - Procedure #1, Procedure #2

Cramping/ Dehydration in doing this stretch and the Fountain of Youth Knee Stretch you may experience cramping in the hamstrings (back of the thigh). If so, you should do the hamstring stretch (to follow) before doing the Anterior Tibialis Stretch.

Video Demonstration of Anterior Tibialis Stretch for Dorsal Foot/ Toe problems

https://www.youtube.com/watch?v=vmRZKydwaAE

Knee

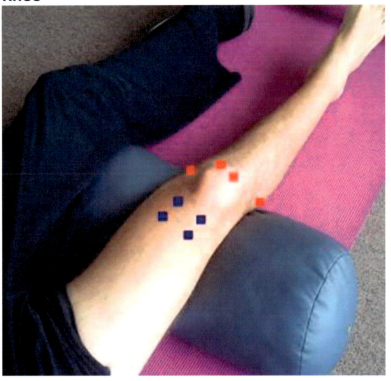

The Quadriceps, Femoris Vastus Lateralis and Vastus Medialis are the targeted muscles for Korean Kinetic Acupuncture's Knee procedure. These are the points represented by the blue squares. The red squares represent acupuncture points Liver 8, Gall Bladder 34, Stomach 35 and the extra points Xi Yan. The blue squares also overlap with acupuncture points Spleen 10 and Stomach 34.

The patella follows a track as the knee is flexed and extended. If there is mal-alignment and uneven tension along the Vastus Lateralis and Medialis the Patella can be pulled off track, resulting in pain and eventual joint deformity.

The KKA Knee procedure is done to even the tension and balance for the Quadriceps and to keep the Patella track correct.

Caution: This procedure should only be done for general knee pain, tendinitis conditions. Do not do this procedure for tears of the ligaments or meniscus of the knee.

Acupuncture Procedure preceding KKA

Before the Korean Kinetic Procedure is performed the licensed acupuncturist can insert Stomach 35 and the extra points Xi Yan up to .5- 1 cun depth in the knee flexed position. Remove these points before beginning KKA. Points Liver 8 and GB 34 can be left in during the KKA knee procedure. Like the KKA Kinetic Shoulder technique, these acupuncture points are not muscle centric but in line with the traditional theories and constructs of Acupuncture, which is to open up channel blockage and obstruction.

KKA Procedure Knee

Patient is lying supine with knee flexed and supported underneath by pillow or cushion.

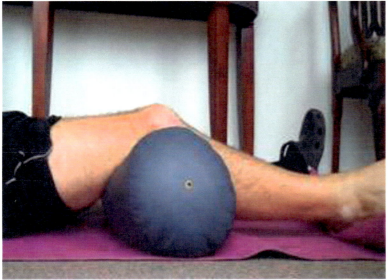

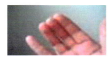

1. Find the trigger point, knotted areas on the Quadriceps Lateral and Medial muscles.
- Massage in a distal to proximal direction with the three middle fingers firmly pressed against the patient's Quadriceps.

2. Insert needles into trigger point areas (superficial .1-.3 cun).

3. Test patient comfort level with needles by moving the knee in flexion and extension.   Adjust the needle outward if discomfort. Watch for dimples surrounding the needle insertion area during movement. Dimple areas may indicate discomfort, adjust the needle outward.

4. Patient comfort with the needles has been assured with a test movement of the knee.

Kinetic Movement #1 for Knee

The practitioner holding the patient at the ankle and supporting at the knee, gently rocks the knee in a lateral and medial direction at the same time as moving the knee in flexion/ extension, up and down. The gentle rocking motion in the lateral / medial plane can be achieved by the practitioners grip at the ankle.

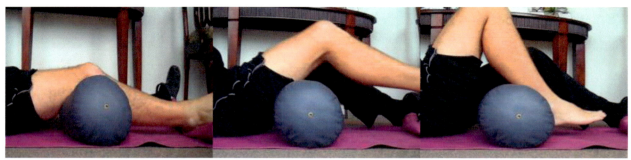

Practitioner gently rocks knee in flexion / extended motion.

Begin KKA Isometric Resistance for Knee

Using the different levels of flexion and extension (no longer gently rocking the knee) the practitioner instructs the patient to extend the lower leg against the practitioner resistance (practitioner resistance at grip point of dorsal ankle foot). By extending the lower leg the quadriceps contract. Resistance doesn't allow for movement of the lower leg so the quadriceps will stretch and balance in lieu of extending the leg.

*The patient should not be lifting from the hips which they may try to flex, to move the lower leg. Be watchful that only the lower leg is being extended, that only the quadriceps are the muscles being fired.

**KKA's Isometric Resistance treatment should be done at differing levels of the knee flexion position. In the three panel picture above the isometric resistance can be performed at each of these levels with the patient trying to extend their lower leg against practitioner resistance.

To the practitioner's count of four the patient tries to extend their lower leg against the resistance of the practitioner. At "four" the patient is instructed to "relax". The practitioner either repeats the procedure at the same level or moves the knee to a different level of flexion.

The exercise is repeated 5- 10 times. After the procedure has been performed needles may either be removed or retained depending on the practitioner's choice for following therapy.

Treatment Plan Triangle for Knee Pain

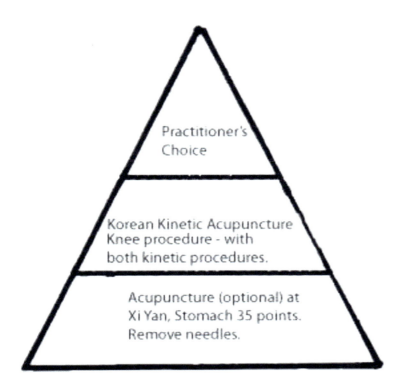

Video Demonstration of Knee Procedure

https://www.youtube.com/watch?v=s4ZH5PKE88I

Patient Self Stretches for Knee Pain (excerpt taken from "Fountain of Youth Stretching" by Dr. Evan Mahoney.

Fountain of Youth Knee Stretch Technique
*You can do the Korean Kinetic Acupuncture Technique with this exercise. With needle placement at Spleen 10, Stomach 34 and ashi points of spleen/ stomach channel on quadriceps. Have the patient flex the knee as fully and comfortably before inserting needles, following with isometric stretch.

Lift your foot up behind you as close and snug to the butt as possible. Leg may be unable to flex fully. Stop when there is pain or resistance. You will feel the stretch of the quadriceps.

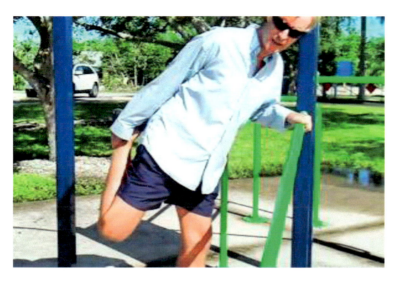

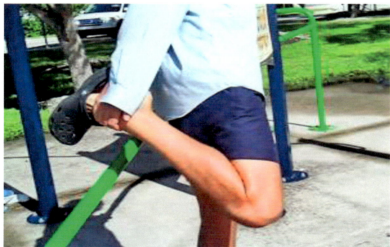

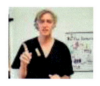 # Add Isometric Stretch

Push the foot against your hand as the knee is in this flexed position. Resist the movement of the foot with your hand.

The Quadriceps contract to extend the foot. When we resist the extension with our hand the foot will not move. The only outcome is that the Quadriceps will stretch.

In the picture above I am pushing my foot and leg down against my right hand. My right hand is resisting that motion. Thereby I end up stretching my quadriceps.

Stretch Knees at different levels (particularly if there is difficulty bringing leg and foot all the way back). By stretching the knees at different levels you will also notice the stretch along different levels of the Quadriceps muscles. Keep doing the Isometric Component at these different levels.

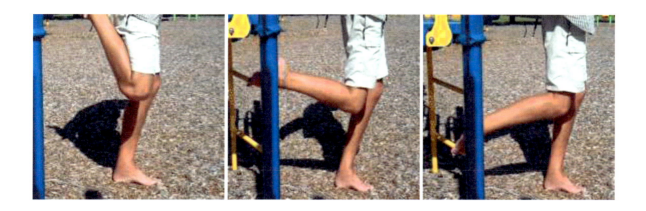

Lower Back and Hip Joint Pain

Any treatment involving Lower Back and Hip Joint Pain will involve VST acupuncture. It is usually the first choice for treatment. The VST procedure for lower back pain is described in the companion book "VST Acupuncture: Capstone and Credentials". The Korean Kinetic Acupuncture Procedure for the Piriformis muscles starts upon the Piriformis and then continues as part of regular VST. VST for Lower Back Pain is done on the patient in the prone position.

Following VST is the mobilization technique Therapeutic Lumbar Technique (TLT) which involves two procedures. The first is a quick needle insertion and withdrawal into the Quadratus Lumborum followed by a mobilization procedure (which will not be presented in these materials).

For troubles at the hip joint and Iliotibial (IT) Band (Tensor Fasciae Latae) VST is performed first, then TLT, followed by the KKA procedure for the hip.

To finish the treatment for Lower Back and Hip Joint Pain I will introduce the Kinetic Decompression Back Stretch which I created but is derived from and is the provenance of acupuncture and oriental medicine.

A word on VST acupuncture for lower back pain

VST for lower back pain will essentially be a practitioner's choice. I find that general acupuncture procedures using traditional acupuncture points along the Urinary Bladder, Gall Bladder, and Ashi points upon the Gluteus Muscles in the prone position are sufficient, in line with TLT and the Kinetic Decompression Stretch to follow.

Piriformis Muscle for Lower Back and Hip Joint (excerpt from "Fountain of Youth Stretching")

The Piriformis is an agonist muscle for external rotation of the hips (and abduction). Meaning, as demonstrated in the picture below when the hips flare out like a frogs, the Piriformis is fully contracted. In order to stretch the Piriformis Muscle we must do the opposite which is to internally rotate the hips.

The Piriformis contracts to initiate external rotation of the hip.

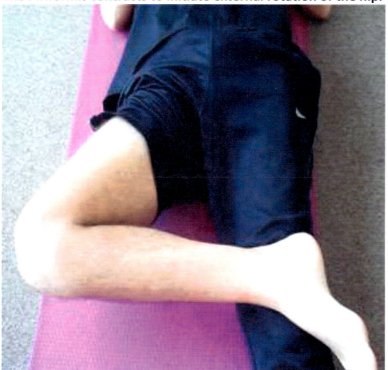

Normal Range of Motion for External Hip Rotation is 45 degrees

My hips are externally rotated.
My Piriformis contracts to
externally rotate my hips. In order
to stretch my Piriformis, I will have to
do the opposite of this, which is to
internally rotate my hips.

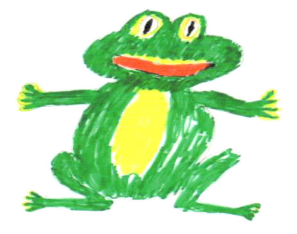

Internal Rotation of the Hip (standing position)

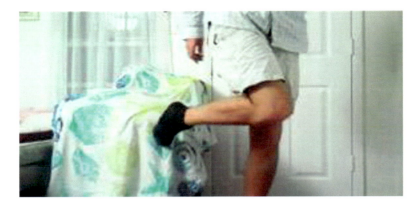

Internal Rotation of the Hip (lying face down). My right hip is internally rotated.

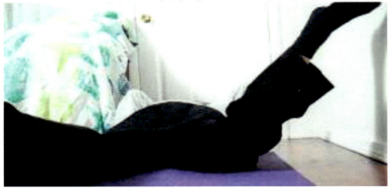

Piriformis is stretched - Normal Internal Range of motion of the hip is 40 degrees.

The Piriformis originates from the anterior sacrum and greater sciatic notch of the ilium and inserts to the Greater Trochanter of the Femur. It external rotates (and abducts) the hip. The Piriformis is located about midlevel of the Gluteus Muscles, halfway between the posterior iliac crest and the lower buttocks.

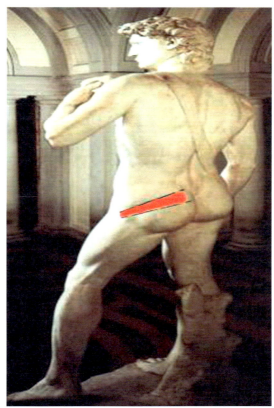

General Location of the Piriformis Muscle

Two types of sciatica.

1. Bulging discs of the vertebrae are the most commonly referred type of sciatic pain. This usually presents with severe at the lumbar vertebrae followed by a track of pain going down lateral hip to legs and feet. This type of sciatic pain is usually constant 24/7 with little positional relief.

2. **Piriformis Syndrome is a peripheral impingement of the Sciatic Nerve (meaning the nerve is being impinged outside of the Spinal Column).** As the Sciatic Nerve travels south from the spinal cord it passes through (in a foramen) or adjacent to the Piriformis Muscle located in the mid to lower gluteus region. The Piriformis can become tight, sticky, and short due to trigger point pathology. As it shortens it impinges on the Sciatic Nerve triggering Sciatic like pain.

   Piriformis Syndrome can be distinguished from a spinal disc problem by the following. Pirifomis Syndrome pain originates from the gluteus region (not the spine, in many cases the patient may not have any pain at lumbar vertebrae) and tracks down the back of the thigh, sometimes going to leg and foot. The radiating pain of Piriformis syndrome may be intermittent with periods and positions of being 'on or off'. Positional relief may be found between sitting, standing, or sleeping.

   Piriformis Syndrome frequently affects the elderly and those who have been sitting in prolonged periods of time. Travel, road trips, and sitting in chairs that pinch at the buttocks can cause Piriformis Syncrome.

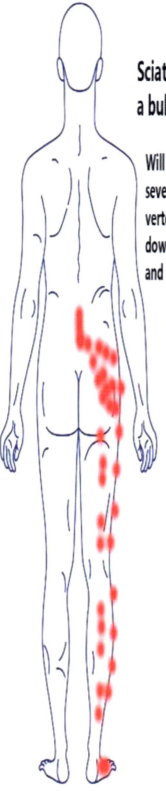

Sciatica from a bulging disc.

Will present with severe pain at lumbar vertebra and tracks down lateral side of leg and foot.

Usually affects younger people.

Pain is usually constant, severe, with no positional relief to be found.

Hurts, walking, sitting, and sleeping.

Sciatica from Piriformis Syndrome

May have no pain at Lumbar Vertebra.

Pain tracks from the mid to lower buttocks down the back of the thigh. May radiate to lateral side of lower leg to foot.

Pain may be bilateral.

Pain may be intermittent, with positional relief found.

Happens frequently to elderly people. Or those who have recently travelled on long road trips. Or from sitting in a chair that compresses lower buttocks.

KKA Piriformis Procedure #1 and #2

KKA Piriformis #1.

Patient is lying prone on the table.

1. Insert needles along the line of the patients Piriformis muscle starting with acupoint Gall Bladder 30 and palpation of trigger points within the triangular area from the Greater Trochanter of the Hip to the Sacrum. (Insert from .5 - 1.5 cun).

2. On the side of the Piriformis Muscle being worked upon, lift the patient's lower leg up so the knee is flexed at 90 degrees. Test patient comfort level with needles by externally rotating the hip (pushing the leg laterally up to 40 degrees. This is internal rotation of the hip, stretching the Piriformis. Adjust the needle outward if discomfort. Watch for dimples surrounding the needle insertion area during movement. Dimple areas may indicate discomfort, adjust the needle outward.

3. Patient comfort with the needles has been assured with a test movement of the Hip and Piriformis.

Begin Isometric Resistance

With the practitioner holding the leg and hip in internal rotation position (the knee is flexed at 90 degrees) the patient is instructed to externally rotate the hip (push the leg medially) against the resistance of the practitioner. The practitioner's resisting hand is placed on the inner ankle and foot while the other hand stabilizes the patients opposite hip on the table (this helps to isolate action to only the contraction of the Piriformis).

To the practitioner's count of four the patient tries to medially push the leg against the resistance of the practitioner. At "four" the patient is instructed to "relax". The practitioner returns the leg to the internally rotated position either at 40 degrees or as far as the patient is comfortable with.

The exercise is repeated 5- 10 times. Keep needles retained after KKA procedure. Continue on with VST acupuncture or Practitioners Choice acupuncture.

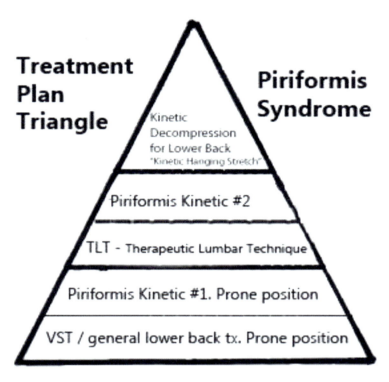

Video Demonstration #1 of Piriformis Procedure. Filmed at Florida State Oriental Medical Association Conference, Fort Lauderdale 2021.

Part II – Kinetic Acupuncture and Piriformis Syndrome
https://youtu.be/MIcm1WSS0HM

Progression of steps in treating Piriformis Syndrome.

1. Bottom position. Local acupuncture (VST), pts along UB channel, etc... Done passively in prone position.
2. Kinetic #1 in prone position. Isometric stretch with hip placed in internal rotation.
3. Not shown in video. Quick Acupuncture into Psoas / Quadratus Lumborum followed by manual back stretch.
4. Kinetic #2. Shown in video
5. Not shown in video. Decompression stretches of back

Video Demonstration #2 of Piriformis Procedure

https://www.youtube.com/watch?v=DoM8NB0OvHU

Piriformis Kinetic Acupuncture Technique #2.

In the treatment plan triangle above this technique comes after Piriformis Kinetic technique #1, local acupuncture (VST or otherwise) to the back, and the Therapeutic Lumbar Technique. After these procedures are performed is when Piriformis #2 is done. This technique is not shown in the treatment plan triangle above.

Post Script: Most of the time I do not do technique #1 anymore (occasionally). I go straight to Piriformis #2 technique, which is as follows. This stretch can be done with or without needles. Patient is lying supine. Position them in the Piriformis stretch (pictured below). In the picture we are stretching the patient's left side piriformis, which is where the needles are placed. After positioning the patient in the stretch position, the practitioner will insert the needles.

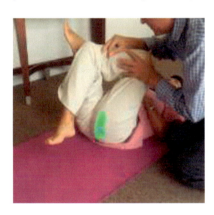

Kinetic Acupuncture for Piriformis Syndrome using Isometric Stretch.

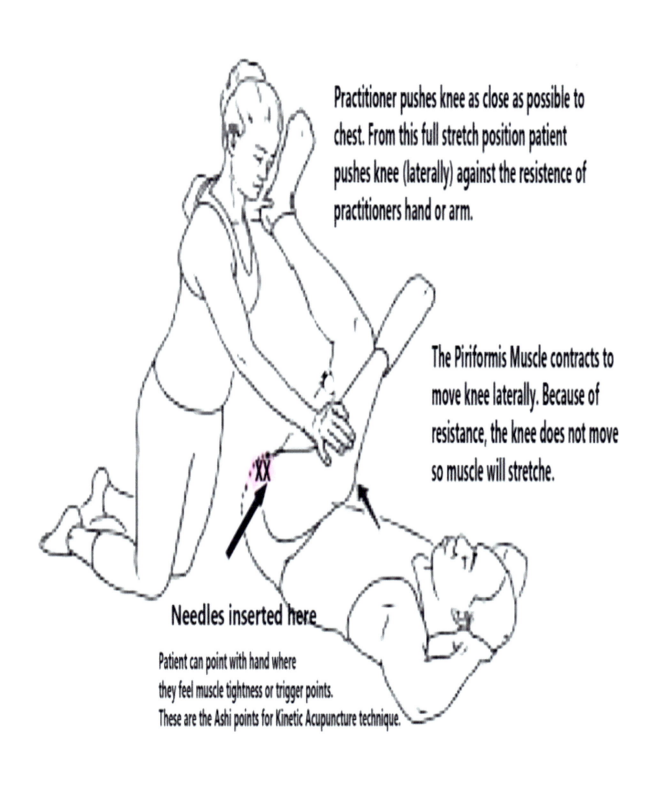

Practitioner pushes knee as close as possible to chest. From this full stretch position patient pushes knee (laterally) against the resistence of practitioners hand or arm.

The Piriformis Muscle contracts to move knee laterally. Because of resistance, the knee does not move so muscle will stretche.

XX

Needles inserted here

Patient can point with hand where they feel muscle tightness or trigger points. These are the Ashi points for Kinetic Acupuncture technique.

In order to assist with needle placement the practitioner can ask the patient to point where the muscle is tight. They will point to the area surrounding the piriformis muscle, lower glutues, and possible upper hamstring. This area marked in the picture above is where the needles are placed.

Practitioner then pushes knee as close to the chest as possible. From this full stretch position patient pushes their knee (without using their hands) laterally against the practitioners hand or arm. This is an isometric stretch. We are placing Piriformis in full stretch. From full stretch patient contracts Piriformis (by pushing knee laterally), because of resistance by practitioner, the knee will not move. Doing this will stretch the Piriformis Muscle.

Immediate results should be expected with this Kinetic Acupuncture treatment of Piriformis Syndrome.

Note: This same stretch can also be done in the sitting position (without needles).

Safety: The above picture demonstrates the location with clothing. Do not needle through the clothing. It is dangerous (particularly with movement) and counter to clean needle technique. Do not needle through clothing.

IT Band (Tensor Fasciae Latae) for Hip Joint

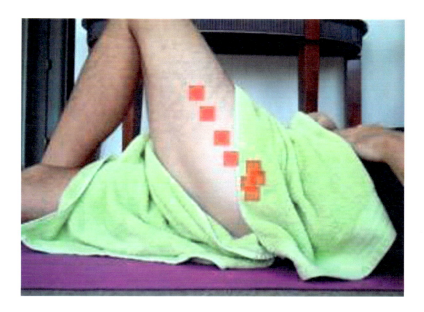

This is the position which the Korean Kinetic Acupuncture IT Band/ Hip Joint procedure is performed in. Notice the left leg crosses over the right knee. The left hip is internally stretching the tissues of the IT Band.

KKA with Isometric Resistance

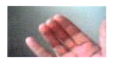

In the position above. Patient supine with their knee flexed and leg crossed over the opposite knee. *Needles may be inserted before crossing patients foot over opposite knee.

1. Find the trigger point, knotted areas of the hip and IT Band
- Massage in a proximal to distal direction (from hip to knee) with the three middle fingers firmly pressed against the patient's IT Band.

2. Insert needles into trigger point areas of Hip and IT Band (superficial .1-.3 cun).

3. Test patient comfort level with needles by moving the patient's knee in a medial and lateral direction (external / internal rotation of the hip). Adjust the needle outward if discomfort. Watch for dimples surrounding the needle insertion area during movement. Dimple areas may indicate discomfort, adjust the needle outward.

4. Patient comfort with the needles has been assured with a test movement of the hip and IT Band.

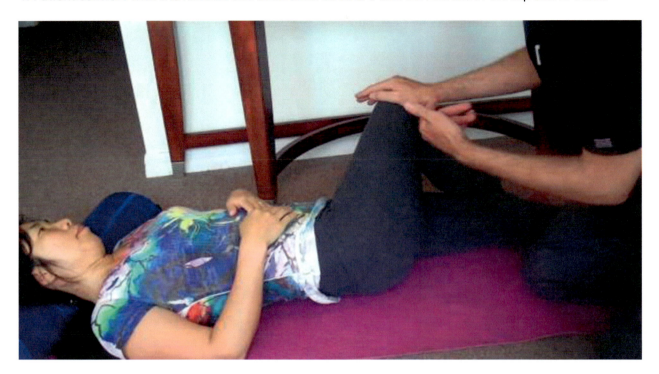

Begin Isometric Resistance

Starting in the position positioned above. The practitioner pushes against the lateral side of the knee to further interiorly rotate the hip as far as the patient is comfortable with. At the furthest point of the stretch the practitioner instructs the patient to push their knee (externally rotate the hip) against the practitioner (practitioner's resisting hand is placed on the lateral part of patients knee).

To the practitioner's count of four the patient tries to laterally push their knee (externally rotate their hip) against the resistance of the practitioner. At "four" the patient is instructed to "relax". The practitioner returns the knee and hip to the interiorly rotated position as far as the patient is comfortable with.

The exercise is repeated 5- 10 times. Remove the needles immediately upon the last isometric resistance stretch.

Treatment Plan Triangle for Lower Back Pain / IT Band Hip Joint

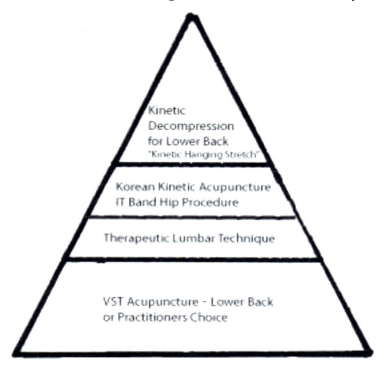

Kinetic
Decompression
for Lower Back
"Kinetic Hanging Stretch"

Korean Kinetic Acupuncture
IT Band Hip Procedure

Therapeutic Lumbar Technique

VST Acupuncture - Lower Back
or Practitioners Choice

Video Demonstration of Hip IT Band Procedure

https://www.youtube.com/watch?v=sBrW9g1vvP0

Therapeutic Lumbar Technique (TLT)

Procedure #1- Needling of the Quadratus Lumborum Muscle Trigger Point

Mapping Location Point - Midpoint between 10th rib and ASIS

Insertion point - Same Level as UB 24, 2 Cun lateral to Midline. Obliquely/ Superficial 1.5 - 2 Cun
Needle towards spine. Do not Angle needle in anterior direction towards internal organs.

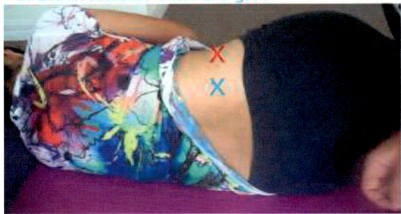

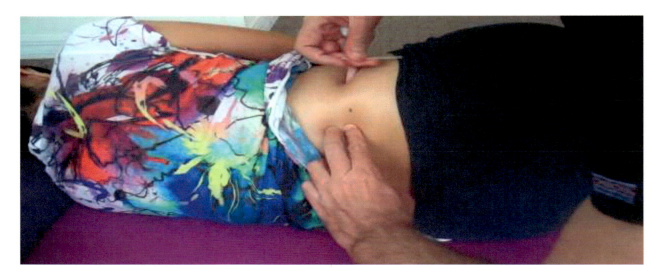

TLT Procedure #2 - will not be demonstrated here.

Video Demonstration of TLT #1 - Quadratus Lumborum

https://www.youtube.com/watch?v=ggLmkKnQ_IE&feature=youtu.be

Kinetic Decompression Stretch for Lower Back aka "Kinetic D - Hanging Back Stretch"

This is a practice and procedure derived wholly from acupuncture by acupuncturist for use with acupuncture. This works best after acupuncture has been performed, which makes the body and muscles more relaxed and pliable for this stretch.

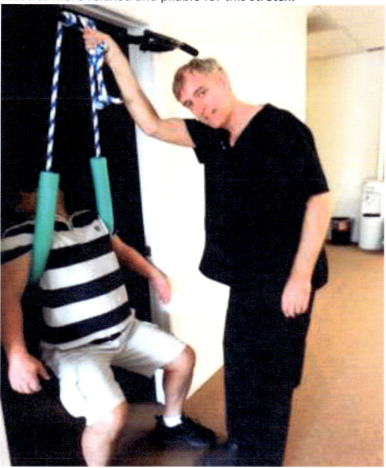

Genesis of the Kinetic D Hanging Back Stretch

During my doctorate clinical training at Samra Acupuncture Center's specialty pain management clinic we performed our Kinetic Acupuncture Lower Back procedure. This is briefly described in the Samra Brochure under the Mobility Plus chapter. Needles would be inserted into acupuncture points on the elbows, feet, neck, and lower back. The patient would then be instructed to do a march while the needles were in place. The march entailed swinging the opposite arm as the opposite leg stepped up high. The head was held high and the back straight. The patient was instructed to imagine a piece of string pulling them up to the sky from the Du 16 acupoint as they did their march.

Sometimes in the more difficult cases the patient had to be supported by two of us in order to do the march. You will see a picture of this in the bottom right hand corner of the brochure page. With a practitioner holding up the patient from underneath each shoulder, they would essentially lift the patient up as they did the march around the clinic.

Inside Samra Acupuncture Center

At Samra Acupuncture Center, we take a contemporary approach to a 2000-year-old discipline to pr

Contemporary Diagnostic Tools

Unlike most acupuncture clinics which rely on questionnaires as their diagnostic tools, Samra Acupuncture Center utilizes state-of-the-art Magnetic Resonance Imaging (MRI), Nerve Conduction Velocity (NCV), and Digital X-Ray imaging to help us accurately pinpoint the origin of our patients' symptoms. We believe this is a crucial part of the acupuncture process, not only because it provides the clearest diagnoses, but it also rules out any life-threatening conditions which might require immediate medical intervention. At Samra Acupuncture Center, medical doctors, chiropractors and acupuncturists all work together, so that the patients' diagnoses and care are viewed from a comprehensive perspective.

Mobility + Acupuncture

"Keep your arms swinging, one-two, one-two, and one-two," leads the instructor as a young man performs what appears to be a formal and vigorous military march. This man is not in training for the army. He is being treated for back pain. If you look closely, you can see that he has barely visible acupuncture needles in his arms and legs. This is part of Samra Acupuncture Center's 'Mobility plus Acupuncture'. This unique treatment of needles and movement has helped alleviate severe and acute pain in many of our patients. Most patients experience immediate and extreme relief.

MRI Image

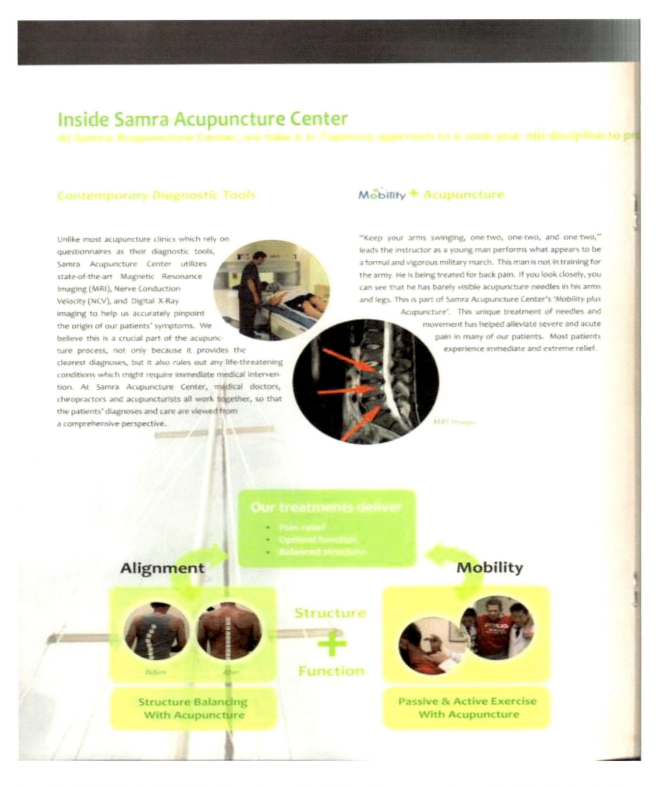

Our treatments deliver
- Pain relief
- Optimal function
- Balanced structure

Alignment

Mobility

Structure

+

Function

Before   *After*

Structure Balancing With Acupuncture

Passive & Active Exercise With Acupuncture

In my book "Eliminate Back Pain - Hang From a Tree" I describe my experience of getting back pain at the beginning of my internship with Samra Acupuncture Center and noted the difficulty of me at 6'2'' having to stoop low in order to lift the patient up and walk them around the clinic.

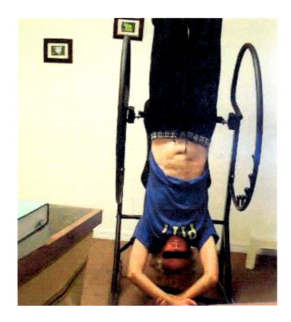

We also used the inversion table as part of our service and which I used to great benefit during my internship. The inversion does two things, both of which can be accomplished with the Kinetic Decompression Lower Back Stretch.

1. It creates separation between the vertebrae
2. It stretches the lower back muscles

By hanging upside down it juxtaposes the constant compression from gravity upon the back in the upright postures.

Later when I moved to Florida and again had a return of severe sciatica with slight foot drop I used this principle of elevation and inversion to create the simple and straight forward "Eliminate Back Pain - Hang from a Tree Back" stretches.

It would be impossible for me to elevate and support patients singlehandedly like we did in Los Angeles, so I created the Kinetic Decompression Lower Back Stretch tool.

Kinetic Decompession Lower Back Stretch Tool
Comprised of three items.
1. A pull up bar/ chin up bar (or tree limb) to stretch from.
2. 12 - 15 feet of rope (Nylon). One half to three quarter inch diameter.
3. Swimming noodle 2-3 inch diameter.

Thread rope through the swimming noodle and tie knots at the end for grip handling.

Instructions on how to use.
Caution: Do not exceed the weight restrictions of the bar you are using. To more easily hold the weight of the patient wrap the rope 2- 3 times around the bar. Ensure the strength of the rope. Ensure patient comfort, especially with the shoulders. Use with caution or do not use if the patient

has any history of neck or shoulder injury or damage. Concern for the shoulders is of the utmost importance.

1. With the patient standing under the bar and facing the practitioner. Place the swimming noodle under the patient's shoulders. Wrap the loose ends of the rope 2-3 times around the bar.*
2. **Caution the patient about shoulder comfort. If pain or discomfort stand up immediately.**
3. Have patient bend their knees and walk their feet in front of them. Assuming the posture in picture one of this chapter.
4. Patient's feet should always be touching the ground.
5. Instruct the patient to relax the muscles from their belly button down and let the weight of gravity pull the lower back down.
6. Discourage patient from swinging or rocking while doing the stretch, they should remain still as they relax the back.
7. Hold the position for 10 seconds
8. When the patient stands up, have them walk in place lifting their legs up as high as possible.
9. Assess the patient.
10. Repeat this exercise 3-5 times. Initially the muscles will resist the stretch. Upon repeating of the stretch the muscles understand better and begin to stretch better.
11. Instruct the patient in the self stretches of the "Eliminate Back Pain - Hang From a Tree" which is comprised of two stretches. One particularly beneficial for the Psoas Muscle.

*Based upon the double block principle in sailing. The rope passes once, twice, or greater through the block. This allows for the easy lifting of greater heavy weights.

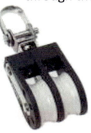

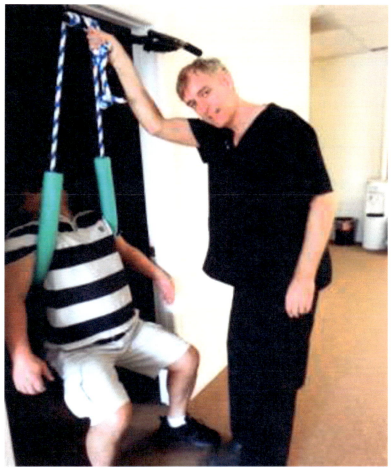

Notice the double wrap around the bar? I'm able to hold the patient up with one hand. Patient's legs are brought forward.

The Kinetic Decompression Stretch for Lower Back allows for a variety of other hip joint mobilization techniques. Please refer to "Eliminate Back Pain - Hang From a Tree" and "Fountain of Youth Stretch" series for other possibilities with the Kinetic Decompression Stretch for Lower Back aka "Kinetic D Hanging Back Stretch".

Video Demonstration of Kinetic Decompression of the Lower Back aka "Kinetic D Hanging Back Stretch"

https://www.youtube.com/watch?v=wNjkp_5zU2w

After the Kinetic Decompression Stretch we teach our patients to hang from a pull up bar. This is my dad at 85 years old doing a Psoas Muscle Stretch with decompression. To see more please read my book "Eliminate Back Pain, Hang from a Tree." We recommend this as a multi time daily stretch to keep our patient's backs healthy for the rest of their lives.

Caution in doing this stretch for people with shoulder injuries and rotator cuff tear history.

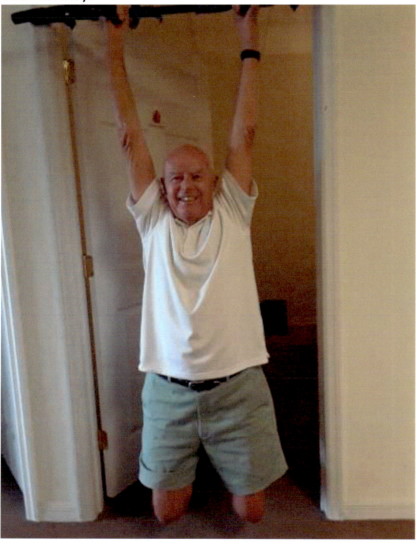

Appendix A - Solution Focused Approach and the Choi Progression Analysis Chart.

Prognosis = Forward Knowing

In my opinion the highest indication of skill by a practitioner is the ability to make a prognosis and stick by it with accurate results.   Dr. Choi emphasized this point to me in one of our impromptu lunchtime lectures. "To correctly make a prognosis will instill confidence of the patient in you" he told me.

With Solution Focused Approach this forward knowing not only applies to prognosis but to the progression and order of therapy, as indicated in the Treatment Plan Triangle. In therapy it becomes a conversation with the patient and their response to Kinetic Acupuncture which many times is expected to yield instant results (according to Choi Progression Analysis Chart). If results are not satisfactory one must look at the next link in the kinetic chain.

Sometimes the patient may lead the practitioner astray. They may come in and say "I have sciatic pain" and point to their lower back and it leads you the practitioner to assume this is a disc related issue of the lower back. When in fact it may be sciatic of the Piriformis syndrome.   So initially you follow the lower back protocol foregoing Piriformis, until you discover results are not satisfactory. Upon exploration you may discover that it is Piriformis syndrome, or maybe it is one further link down the chain and is hamstring muscle spasm.

The same situation may present in radiculopathy due to cervical degenerative disc disease. Only to discover that it is a peripheral nerve impingement at the Teres Major. The orderly step by step progression treatment plan triangle and prognosis model are examples of knowledgeable Solution Focused Approach.

Here is the Choi Progression Analysis Chart - from "Saam Acupuncture: Advanced Combinations" - Book #2 in the "Saam Medical Meditation" series.

Choi Progression Analysis Chart [xxxvi]

The Choi Progression Analysis Chart is used for purposes of making a prognosis of musculoskeletal pain of the lower back (and most other types of pain). It is based upon the therapeutic procedures of Korean Kinetic Acupuncture. It gives the therapist skills to predict the outcome of their treatment and the recommended duration of treatment.

Choi's Progression Analysis Chart

	Intensity of Pain	Getting Better	
	A		B
	Acute - Sub Acute (up to 6 months)		*Chronic*
	C	Getting Worse	D

Duration of complaint

Explanation of Category

Category A   **"Celebrate, Victory is Near"**

Acute Stage / Getting better – This is the most positive of prognosis. This generally refers to muscle strains/ sprains with sudden onset. The patient was lifting or twisting something when they got a sudden sharp pain.

Therapy should be limited between 1 – 3 times within two weeks before problem is resolved.

Category B   "Nearing the End of a Painful Time"

Chronic Stage / Getting Better - This can cautiously be considered a positive prognosis. This generally refers to the end stage of a disc related problem. Disc problems should resolve themselves spontaneously within six months. Patient can resume to normal function. The clearing of inflammation to the pinched nerve, and the rebuilding of channel connections makes for a longer term therapy between 10 -15 times within two months.

Category C   "What are we dealing with here?"

Acute stage/ Getting Worse – A diagnosis is essential for this category. We need to rule out between a sprain /strain, disc problem, tumor, arthritis, or another problem. The patient intake and examination shall lead one to a diagnosis, further confirmed by an MRI or Xray. The diagnosis will determine the therapeutic plan. If it is a sprain / strain see category A. If it is a disc problem see category B.

Category D   "In for the Long Haul"

Chronic stage/ Getting Worse – This generally applies to disc patients with multiple episodes, spinal stenosis, back operations, arthritis, and other serious conditions. This is the poorest of prognosis, and is difficult to treat. This will require long term therapy, over 20 times for up to six months. Possibility that patient may achieve only minimal, temporary results, or relapse after improvement.

Footnotes from "Dry Needle Technique and Arguments for the Defense of Acupuncture" Capstone project

i The normal range of motion degrees are taken from http://www.chiro.org/forms/romchiro.html

ii The normal range of motion degrees are taken from http://www.chiro.org/forms/romchiro.html

iii Lee, Jonghwa, Choi, Hyungsuk, Lee Woongkyung, Ee Dongyup, Vertex Synchronizing Technique Acupuncture (Tensegrity Model Acupuncture), unknown date of publication, Samra University of Oriental Medicine.

iv The normal range of motion degrees are taken from http://www.chiro.org/forms/romchiro.html

v The normal range of motion degrees are taken from http://www.chiro.org/forms/romchiro.html

vi Lee, Jonghwa, Choi, Hyungsuk, Lee Woongkyung, Ee Dongyup, Vertex Synchronizing Technique Acupuncture (Tensegrity Model Acupuncture), unknown date of publication, Samra University of Oriental Medicine.

vii Lee, Jonghwa, Choi, Hyungsuk, Lee Woongkyung, Ee Dongyup, Vertex Synchronizing Technique Acupuncture (Tensegrity Model Acupuncture), unknown date of publication, Samra University of Oriental Medicine.

viii Lee, Jonghwa, Choi, Hyungsuk, Lee Woongkyung, Ee Dongyup, Vertex Synchronizing Technique Acupuncture (Tensegrity Model Acupuncture), unknown date of publication, Samra University of Oriental Medicine.

ix Lee, Jonghwa, Choi, Hyungsuk, Lee Woongkyung, Ee Dongyup, Vertex Synchronizing Technique Acupuncture (Tensegrity Model Acupuncture), unknown date of publication, Samra University of Oriental Medicine.

x Lee, Jonghwa, Choi, Hyungsuk, Lee Woongkyung, Ee Dongyup, Vertex Synchronizing Technique Acupuncture (Tensegrity Model Acupuncture), unknown date of publication, Samra University of Oriental Medicine.

xi Lee, Jonghwa, Choi, Hyungsuk, Lee Woongkyung, Ee Dongyup, Vertex Synchronizing Technique Acupuncture (Tensegrity Model Acupuncture), unknown date of publication, Samra University of Oriental Medicine.

xii Lee, Jonghwa, Choi, Hyungsuk, Lee, Woongkyung Lee, Dongyup. "Vertex Synchronizing Technique Acupuncture (Tensegrity Model Acuppuncture) conference article 2009 Society for Acupuncture Research – Translational Research in Acupuncture: bridging Science, Pracitice and Community (SAR 2010), Chapel Hill, North Carolina March 19-21 2010

xiii Cheng Xinnong (Chief Editor) "Chinese Acupuncture and Moxibustion" page 116, revised edition 1999, Foreign Langauage Press, Beijing China

xiv Cheng Xinnong (Chief Editor) "Chinese Acupuncture and Moxibustion" page 116, revised edition 1999, Foreign Langauage Press, Beijing China

xv David G. Simons, Cardiology and Myofascial Trigger PointsJanet G. Travell's Contribution Tex Heart Inst J. 2003; 30(1): 3–7.

xvi David G. Simons, Cardiology and Myofascial Trigger PointsJanet G. Travell's Contribution

Tex Heart Inst J. 2003; 30(1): 3–7.

xvii Gunn, C Chan, "The Gunn Approach to the Treatment of Chronic Pain, Intramuscular Stimulation for Myofascial Pain of Radiculopathic Origin" Churchill livingstone1996 reprinted 2008 summary page 23

xviii Gunn, c. Chan, "The Gunn Approach to the Treatment of Chronic Pain, Intramuscular Stimulation for Myofascial Pain of Radiculopathic Origin" Churchill livingstone1996 reprinted 2008 pages 6-7

xix Gunn, c. Chan, "The Gunn Approach to the Treatment of Chronic Pain, Intramuscular Stimulation for Myofascial Pain of Radiculopathic Origin" Churchill livingstone1996 reprinted 2008 page 7 xx Gunn, c. Chan, "The Gunn Approach to the Treatment of Chronic Pain, Intramuscular Stimulation for Myofascial Pain of Radiculopathic Origin" Churchill livingstone1996 reprinted 2008. This definition from Preface to Second Editionii.

xxi Gunn, c. Chan, "The Gunn Approach to the Treatment of Chronic Pain, Intramuscular Stimulation for Myofascial Pain of Radiculopathic Origin" Churchill livingstone1996 reprinted 2008 pages 11-12

xxii . Lee, Jonghwa "VST study guide from Samra University lecture"

xxiii . Lee, Jonghwa "VST study guide from Samra University lecture"

xxiv David G. Simons, Cardiology and Myofascial Trigger PointsJanet G. Travell's Contribution

Tex Heart Inst J. 2003; 30(1): 3–7.

xxv Gunn, C Chan, "The Gunn Approach to the Treatment of Chronic Pain, Intramuscular Stimulation for Myofascial Pain of Radiculopathic Origin" Churchill livingstone1996 reprinted 2008 overview page 6

xxvi Gunn, C Chan, "The Gunn Approach to the Treatment of Chronic Pain, Intramuscular Stimulation for Myofascial Pain of Radiculopathic Origin" Churchill livingstone1996 reprinted 2008 summary page 23

xxvii Lee, Jonghwa, Choi, Hyungsuk, Lee, Woongkyung Lee, Dongyup. "Vertex Synchronizing Technique Acupuncture (Tensegrity Model Acuppuncture, abstract) conference article 2009 Society for Acupuncture Research – Translational Research in Acupuncture: bridging Science, Pracitice and Community (SAR 2010), Chapel Hill, North Carolina March 19-21 2010

xxviii Lee, Jonghwa, Choi, Hyungsuk, Lee, Woongkyung Lee, Dongyup. "Vertex Synchronizing Technique Acupuncture (Tensegrity Model Acuppuncture, page 3-4 Conference article 2009 Society for Acupuncture Research – Translational Research in Acupuncture: bridging Science, Pracitice and Community (SAR 2010), Chapel Hill, North Carolina March 19-21 2010

xxix Verdier, Renee, "Animal Architecture: Buckminster Fuller's Tensegrity" Renee Verdier Blog. 3/2/09 www.realitysandwich.com/animal_architecture_buckminster_fuller_tensegrity

xxx Verdier, Renee - ibid

xxxi Tensegrity picture from http://www.anatomytrains.com/explore/tensegrity/explained
http://www.google.com/imgres?imgurl=http://www.anatomytrains.com/uploads/static/Image/Tensegrity_Skelet on_10%3D03.jpg&imgrefurl=http://www.anatomytrains.com/explore/tensegrity/explained&usg=__r3lONqXjWILK XzTRClU3q0Kd0UU=&h=450&w=261&sz=15&hl=en&start=94&zoom=1&tbnid=FQeH_SGGrq8c0M:&tbnh=122&tbn w=78&prev=/images%3Fq%3Dtensegrity%2Bmodel%2Bpictures%26um%3D1%26hl%3Den%26sa%3DX%26rlz%3D1 R2SKPB_enUS391%26biw%3D1180%26bih%3D532%26tbs%3Disch:10%2C2038&um=1&itbs=1&ei=pending&iact=h c&vpx=300&vpy=140&dur=437&hovh=219&hovw=127&tx=98&ty=108&oei=_iXnTITcHIP48AbN9cHXDA&esq=2&p age=6&ndsp=23&ved=1t:429,r:1,s:94&biw=1180&bih=532

xxxii Choi, Hyung Suk, Samra Acupuncture Center brochure page 6, published 2009 by Samra Acupuncture center

xxxiii Lee, Jonghwa, Choi, Hyungsuk, Lee, Woongkyung Lee, Dongyup. "Vertex Synchronizing Technique Acupuncture (Tensegrity Model Acuppuncture) conference article 2009 Society for Acupuncture Research – Translational Research in Acupuncture: bridging Science, Pracitice and Community (SAR 2010), Chapel Hill, North Carolina March 19-21 2010

xxxiv Lee, Jonghwa, Choi, Hyungsuk, Lee, Woongkyung Lee, Dongyup. "Vertex Synchronizing Technique Acupuncture (Tensegrity Model Acuppuncture) conference article 2009 Society for Acupuncture Research – Translational Research in Acupuncture: bridging Science, Pracitice and Community (SAR 2010), Chapel Hill, North Carolina March 19-21 2010

xxxv Lee, Jonghwa "VST study guide from Samra University lecture" pages 2-3 2009

Made in United States
Troutdale, OR
04/06/2025

30366923R00093